Nature Play at Home

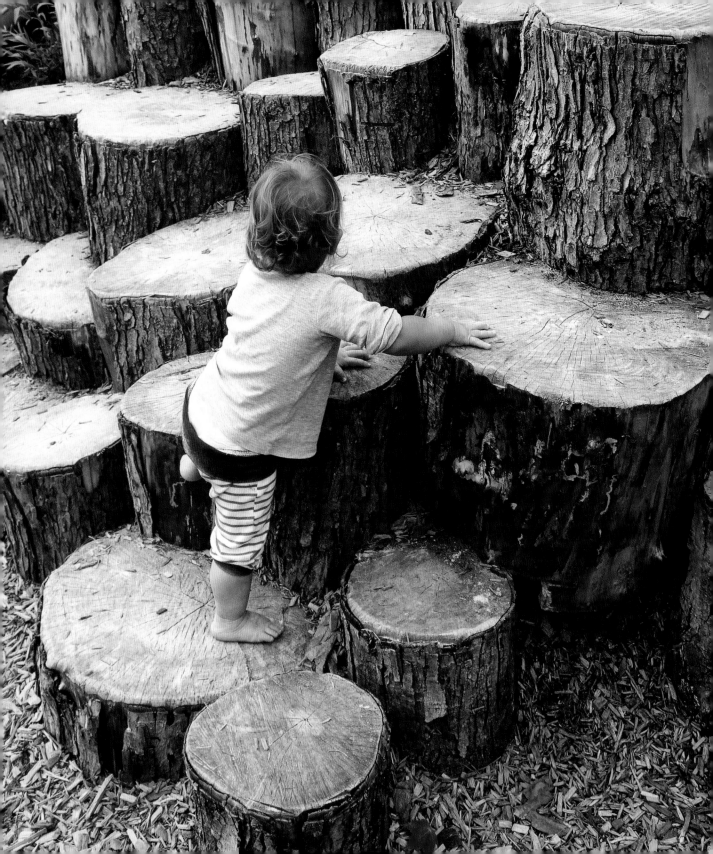

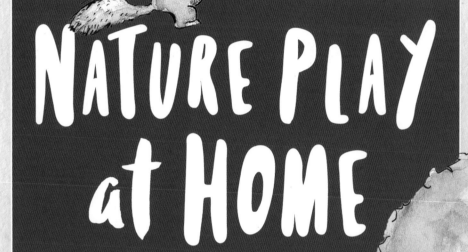

NATURE PLAY at HOME

CREATING **OUTDOOR SPACES** THAT
CONNECT CHILDREN WITH THE **NATURAL WORLD**

NANCY STRINISTE FOUNDER OF EARLYSPACE

ILLUSTRATIONS BY JENNIFER REN

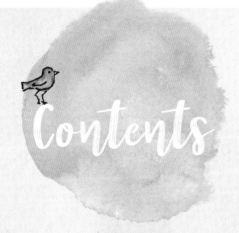

Contents

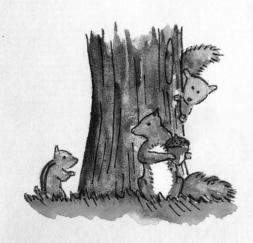

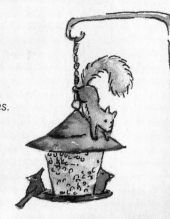

*Dedicated to all my teachers
—both children and adults—
who taught me the power of spaces and places.*

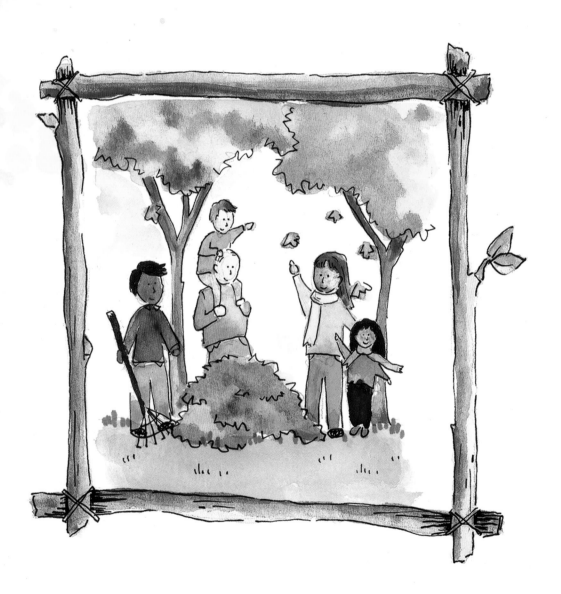

INTRODUCTION

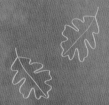

"The key is to understand what nourishes our children and use this awareness to inform every step of the design process."

—from the *Child Care Design Guide*, by Anita Rui Olds

CHILDHOOD HAS CHANGED.

When you think back to your own childhood (especially if you are of a certain age), you probably remember spending a lot of time outdoors, roaming free, climbing trees, building stuff, and mucking in mud.

Children's lives have become more structured and supervised. Many kids spend a great deal of time in front of screens and much less time than past generations playing outside. Academic pressures and parental fears are just two of the reasons for this shift. Depending on where a family lives, fears may be based on real danger outside the door, or created by media that escalates unrealistic worries. Many parents are afraid to allow their children outside unattended, and too busy to accompany them as often as needed. Distance or traffic can make access to play places difficult, which further separates children from these essential experiences of unstructured activity outside in nature.

To illustrate this dilemma, consider a 2007 report by Dr. William Bird, published by Natural England and the Royal Society for the Protection of Birds. It compared four members of a family, each in a different generation, and their outdoor experiences at age 8. When George, the great-grandfather, was 8 years old in 1926, he walked everywhere because his family could not afford a bike for him. He regularly walked six miles on his own to his favorite fishing spot. In 1950, when the grandfather was 8 years old, he walked a mile on his own to play in the woods, and also walked to school. The mother was an 8-year-old in 1979, and was allowed to ride her bike throughout the neighborhood and to the local pool, a half-mile away. Edward, an 8-year-old in 2007, was driven the short distance to school and taken by car to a safe place to ride his bicycle. He was allowed to go about 300 yards to the end of his block on his own, but often didn't enjoy that because there were no other children outside. Edward took piano lessons and skiing lessons and had a trampoline and jungle gym in his yard.

Humans have an innate need to seek connections with nature and other forms of life. E.O. Wilson called this drive biophilia. When this drive is denied, and children don't have the opportunity to form essential relationships with the natural environment, there are consequences for children's physical and mental health and for

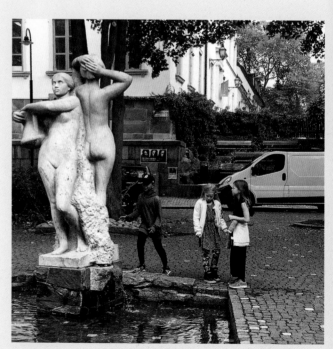

Free-range kids in Stockholm, Sweden, perhaps drawn by the natural elements of water and trees in this park. Seeing children unaccompanied by adults, roaming on their own, stopping to chat and play is a rare sight in American cities today. We've discovered that children losing their outdoor freedom comes at a cost.

their anxiety and stress levels. Thanks to Richard Louv, who gathered all the pieces and first presented them so compellingly in his book *Last Child in the Woods* (2005), we now have a term that describes what many of today's children experience. Louv called it nature deficit disorder, and by naming it, he launched a worldwide movement and a basis for critical conversations.

An exploding body of research tells us that time in nature is crucial to healthy human development. It improves the body's overall health and reduces allergies, anxiety, and symptoms of ADHD. It boosts confidence, creativity, and cooperation as children play. Time in nature also encourages active play, which reduces obesity.

There is even evidence that nearsightedness is reduced and test scores are improved when children spend more time outdoors in nature.

It is heart-wrenching to see the limits placed on play in so many ways and in so many places. Recess has been shortened and is non-existent in some schools. Covenants at condos and in subdivisions limit play to sterile spaces, and parks prohibit tree climbing. But there is, I believe, reason to be encouraged. On many fronts, the pendulum is swinging back.

Across the country and around the world, committed mothers and fathers, along with educators, caregivers, and policymakers, are working to provide more recess and require less sitting time. Many parents have made a conscious decision to reduce scheduled extracurricular activities, wanting their children to spend more time in

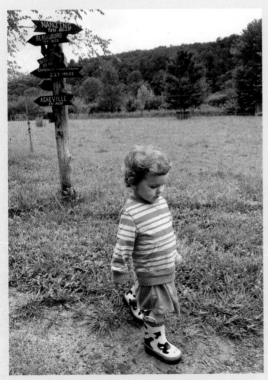

People of all ages need a connection to nature to be happy, healthy, and to think clearly and creatively.

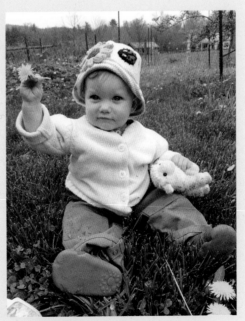

It's never too early to help children discover the natural world around them.

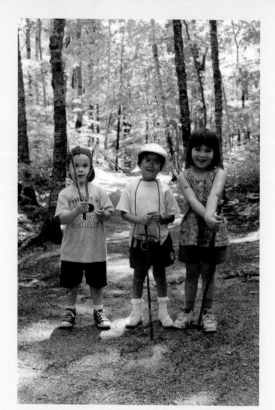

Trails are great for luring young explorers outside.

nature. Families are organizing nature clubs, and there is a growing number of forest schools and adventure playgrounds popping up across the United States.

For me, as a designer in this field for more than thirty years, the swing is evidenced by the growing number of inquiries I get from families, schools, early childhood programs, and municipalities, all looking to provide nearby places where their children can play in nature.

This book is intended as a guide to help you as a parent understand, advocate for, and bring nature play to your neighborhood—whether it is in your local park, your children's schoolyard, common spaces in your community, or your own backyard. I've had the opportunity to create some

wonderful backyard play spaces, working with my crew of top-notch landscape professionals. The cost of a professionally designed space is sometimes out of reach for a young family, but that doesn't mean you can't have a place to play in nature. My hope is to support families in their efforts to create their own natural backyard play spaces. Some families, especially those living in densely built cities, don't have their own backyard to transform, so they turn to shared spaces. I'm often approached by parents who want to make change happen at their child's school or childcare center. Sometimes it is a group of parents who have joined together to form a committee through their PTA or board and want to transform their school's outdoor space. But it can also be a lone parent, who knows the outdoor area at his or her child's school could be better for students, and is determined, despite an initial lack of institutional support, to make change happen.

UNSTRUCTURED TIME

Having abundant unstructured time to explore the outdoors at one's own pace is not a luxury, but an essential element of growing up competent, confident, healthy, and strong. It is our responsibility, as the caretakers of our children's little hearts and spirits, to give our kids plenty of time and opportunities to marvel, to immerse themselves in the power and exhilaration of nature, and to fall in love with the natural world. An aspect of that is beginning to let go of scheduled lessons, teams, and structured activities, to free up the time children need to be able to absorb what nature has to give them. Another piece is bringing nature *to* children, in the places

WORKING FOR THE COMMON GOOD

My client Julie is an attorney who works for justice in her job and in her personal life. Her children had attended the Clarendon Child Care Center in Arlington, Virginia, and she and her kids loved the natural play space there. When her children entered a public school that drew families from across a diverse county, she was surprised by the limited recess time and absence of nature on the playground. She was an involved parent, and volunteering one day in her son's kindergarten class, she had an experience that clarified her purpose. The class was making bird feeders (cardboard dipped in shortening and bird seed) and more than half the class said they lived in apartments and didn't have a tree on which to hang their bird feeder. At that moment, she committed to changing the outdoor space at her children's school. Six years and two beautiful courtyards later, the school is a model for outdoor learning, thanks in large part to Julie's tireless advocacy, fundraising, and hands on the ground. She's written many successful grants (based in part on the bird feeder story), recruited dozens of volunteers, secured donations from the families and the wider community, driven borrowed pickup trucks full of mulch and plants, and spent many days with three devoted master gardeners, including her mom, caring for the courtyards. The Reading Garden and the Art Garden courtyards are two lush oases in this city school, getting children outside among plants, flowing water, and birds and insects. The courtyards are cherished by the teachers, children, and families.

Besides being a landscape designer, I am also a former teacher, and I believe that all children, no matter where they live or go to school, deserve childhoods connected to the wonder of nature. Whether you are working with professionals on a major landscape project at home, doing it yourself on the weekends, or advocating like Julie for transformation in your community, her story proves that you can help bring children closer to nature regardless of where you live.

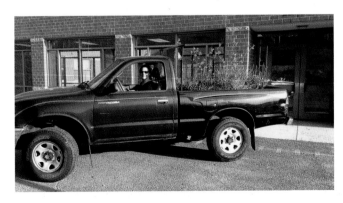

When she discovered that many of her son's kindergarten classmates lacked a place at home to hang a bird feeder, Julie took action to create natural spaces within the schoolyard.

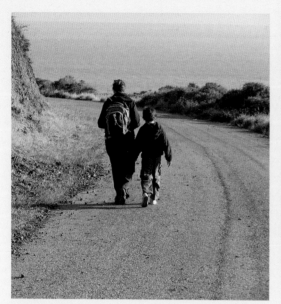

For our well-being, we all need access to wild places. But excursions to places such as shorelines can take planning and work. Nature play near home is close and simple.

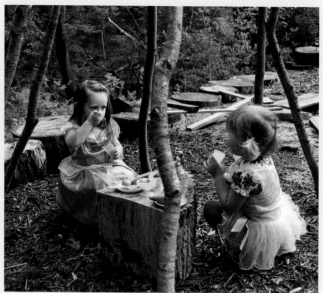

Natural environments are rich catalysts for imaginative play.

where they already spend time—on the school playground, at a local park, and in their own backyards.

WHAT IS A NATURAL PLAY SPACE?

A natural play space incorporates materials such as logs and tree parts, boulders, earth, sand, water, and plants of all kinds, along with evidence of the seasons and the company of wildlife, to create irresistible places for kids to play. Unlike traditional swing sets and play equipment, natural play spaces range from aesthetically beautiful landscapes to wild and messy places, but they invite children from toddlers to teens to venture out and explore nature in a hands-on way.

In creating a natural play space, we have the opportunity to think about engaging all the senses, with fragrance, colors, textures, edibles, and sounds. Elements from and of the earth compose the design palette. Such connections touch children's spirits, and kids are inspired to move, explore, create, and understand.

To create spaces that will work, that will resonate deeply with children, it's helpful to first take a look at where we've been.

A Journey Back in Time

You are no doubt a parent, grandparent, or perhaps a professional who knows and cares about children. We all share another type of expertise. We are all former children. If we search our memories, the child we once were has a tremendous amount to teach us about spaces and places and what was magical. Try this exercise to help you connect with what you knew as a child.

Think back, and find the child inside of you. Picture yourself. Imagine looking down at your little feet, your small arms and hands. Imagine how it felt to be that busy little person. Then remember a favorite spot from your childhood, a special place from anywhere, any time, a place where you might have felt happy, or safe, or content, or free. Remember it. Let your mind take you back there. Think of the details. How it looked. What you could see when you were there. The colors, the light, the objects, the textures. How did it feel? What was above you and below you? Remember the sounds, the smells, the temperature. Think of what you did when you were there, who you were when you were there, and what you liked.

I've recited those words hundreds of times as a guided visualization with parents, educators, students, and colleagues. I love this activity because it transports people out of their practical adult mindsets, which can include a bias toward keeping youngsters clean, dry, and free of bumps and bruises. These memories allow us to reconnect with what was magical early in our lives—a mental framework that sets the stage for designing a great outdoor space for children. I don't believe that "easy to maintain" should be more important than fun and adventure (although of course that feature is worthy of discussion during the process). As you read this book, I hope you will be in a playful state of mind. I hope you will

be able to see the world through the lens of the child you once were.

As you remembered a place from your childhood, was it outside? Were you alone or with friends? Were there adults around? As people share their memories, certain themes emerge again and again, in part because of the evolutionary significance they have to us as a species. See if you agree.

TREES

Many of us have powerful memories of climbing a favorite tree and being up high with a view out of a leafy perch. From that protected vantage point, our primitive ancestors could see predators, but could not be seen. As children, we were not likely worried about being eaten by a saber-toothed tiger, but there was a deep sense of comfort and empowerment that still came from being in that secure and elevated perch. And that made the memory stay with us to adulthood. It is important to remember that humans once climbed trees for safety. As recently as a generation ago, climbing trees wasn't considered dangerous for children; it doesn't have to be now.

ENCLOSURE

Whether it is in a rocky ravine or a cave, in a cluster of shrubs or vines, beneath a tree, or in any sort of built structure, the feeling of being protected and enclosed—from weather, danger, or even too much openness—is tremendously appealing and valuable.

We remember the forts, lean-tos, and tree-houses we built. We even recall the spaces we discovered under a porch or behind a shed. Many of these nests gave us a sense of accomplishment

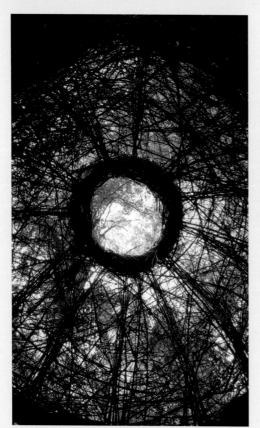

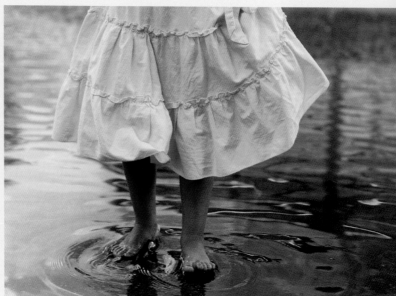

Water play during childhood is often long remembered.

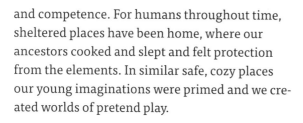

Organic enclosures can make us feel wrapped safely in nature.

and competence. For humans throughout time, sheltered places have been home, where our ancestors cooked and slept and felt protection from the elements. In similar safe, cozy places our young imaginations were primed and we created worlds of pretend play.

HILLS

Terrain can offer the opportunity to experience a new perspective. An elevated, expansive view that allowed us to survey the area, watch for friends or foes, or plan our next destination or activity were all advantages that made the spot atop a hill so valuable to our forebears. Access to

high places helps children understand and monitor their space and the things going on within that space. Traversing level changes and uneven ground (whether they are organic parts of a site or mounds and moguls that have been built) helps children develop stamina and a sense of balance.

WATER

Water is a powerful source of memories. From the expansive ocean to a trickling stream, water has always been key to our survival, and it has a magnetic appeal to children—as our recollections remind us and as we see in children today. Living near the beach, playing on the mossy banks of a woodland stream, or even poking around an urban fountain, the kind of deep engagement that happens around water is universal.

GATHERING

My father-in-law, who grew up in China, often told of a favorite memory from his childhood. He was alone outside in the garden of their house. With a stick, he dug some bamboo shoots. He found an old tin can and some water, built a fire, and cooked the bamboo shoots. This experience was key to his sense of himself as competent and self-sufficient. Many of us have recollections of gathering and pretending to or actually cooking and eating wild food. Perhaps it was snacking in a grandparent's garden or a blueberry patch in a nearby meadow. Our early experiences of finding and gathering food stay with us throughout our lives and connect us to the wild foragers and farmers of the past.

These recurring topics in memories relate to what is sometimes called habitat theory, a framework first put forth by Jay Appleton in the mid-1970s for understanding the meaning and evolutionary significance of common, universal themes. As Jan White and Helen Woolley explain in *Exploring Outdoor Play in the Early Years* (2014), habitat theory says that "preferences for particular landscape features are seen to correspond with an evolutionary and deep-seated psychological drive to ensure that our survival needs are met." As we create spaces that today's children will remember, understanding the appeal of these archetypal elements can inform our designs.

WHAT YOU'LL FIND HERE

This book is a culmination of my passion, my area of expertise, and my life's work: designing sustainable natural play and learning spaces for

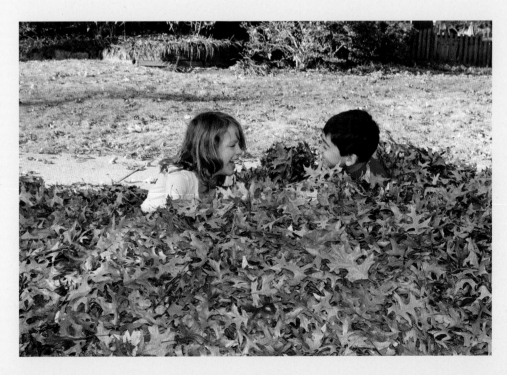

When kids play in a pile of autumn leaves, they literally immerse themselves in nature.

NATURE MAKES US HEALTHIER

In 1997, a seminal study from Sweden led by Patrik Grahn began to quantify the value of children's time in nature. This interdisciplinary research brought together physicians, psychologists, educators, and designers to study and examine nature play from a variety of dimensions. The researchers compared children in so-called traditional Swedish childcare centers, with some asphalt pathways, riding toys, and manufactured play equipment, to children in outdoors-in-all-weather schools, where children and teachers spent the majority of their time outside in nature—meadows, streams, and forests.

By every measure, the school children spending more time in natural environments were doing better. From less illness to lower blood pressure, more upper body strength to the ability to balance on one foot longer, the physical condition of children who spent more time in nature was better. In addition, teachers in these schools spent more time as resources and less time policing student behavior and dealing with conflict.

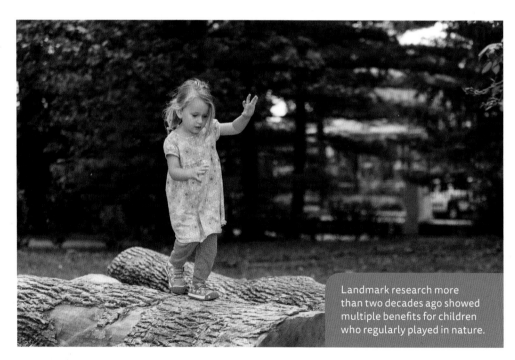

Landmark research more than two decades ago showed multiple benefits for children who regularly played in nature.

children. I have more than thirty years of experience creating inviting, beautiful spaces that connect children to nature, and I am eager to pass along what I've learned. Much of what I offer may feel intuitive, but now science is uncovering the "why." Understanding the significance of nature in human health, and how to address that understanding, is a rapidly advancing field, and each new study tells us more clearly, more specifically, why we can't afford *not* to pay attention.

Whatever your connection to children, if you are searching for ways to balance screen time with time-honored experiences of childhood—playing, exploring, and messing around in nature—I hope to offer some inspiration and answers.

Each chapter addresses a different aspect of what outdoor spaces can be and do, providing a play-based developmental context for the chapter's focus, along with lots of inspiring visuals. There are unique DIY projects that you (yes, you!) can build, as a family or as a neighborhood. My hope is that the process of creating these special places will bring people together with a sense of fun and shared purpose. Throughout, there are recommendations of plants to optimize your efforts: edible plants, plants to stir young imaginations, plants with pickable parts, plants to climb and hide among, plants to shade and shelter, and plants to cushion the ground beneath little feet. We'll also look at the role of native plants in play, habitat, and four-season beauty.

I hope that all these components help you better understand the value of natural play spaces in close proximity to where children live and learn. I hope you and other families feel informed, inspired, and equipped with the practical

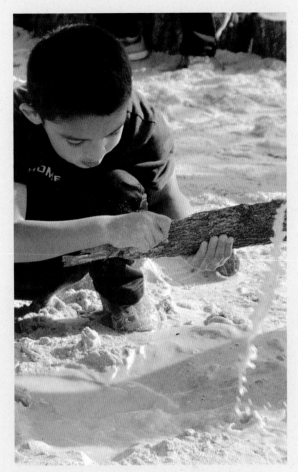

Basic elements such as sand, wood, and water engage developing bodies and minds.

knowledge and resources to begin creating these essential places. And I hope those of you who are parents and grandparents come away convinced that what you remember from childhood is exactly what today's and tomorrow's kids still need—nature nearby, and ample time to play in it freely.

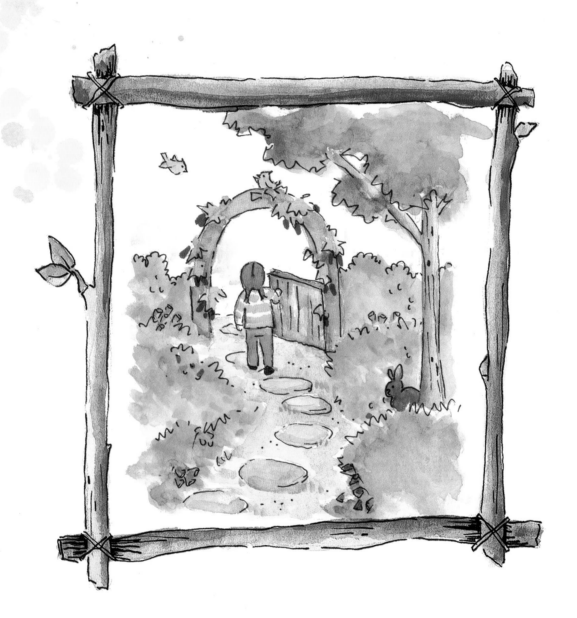

ARRANGING
SPACES

"Natural settings for children's play
that previous generations took for granted must
now be deliberately created."

—from *Nature Play and Learning Places*,
by Robin Moore with Allen Cooper

Spaces speak, especially to children. Just as the soaring ceiling of a cathedral inspires a sense of awe or a candlelit restaurant prompts us to lower our voices, the formality, informality, size, or openness of a space can tell us how to behave. As we create spaces for nature play, it is our responsibility to be mindful and intentional about the messages the space will transmit to children. Spaces for children can be organized and designed to honor and communicate respect for them. What's needed is to build with an understanding of a child's development—and with joy and a sense of fun.

ENTRYWAYS

Creating an enticing, child-oriented entry is our opportunity to invite children into a natural play space, by indicating to them that the area they are about to enter is special. We want the entry to say "this is a place for you" and "come in, there are good, interesting things happening here." To create an enchanting main entry, it is important to think about the *experience* of entering the space and make it more than just the functional step of transitioning from one area to another. Details are important. An entryway is an

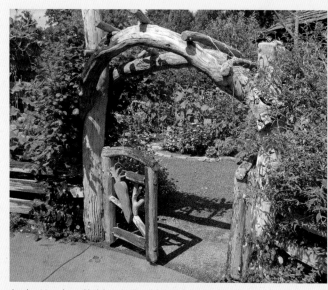

At the Hershey Children's Garden in the Cleveland Botanical Garden, this whimsical arch and gate tell kids that this is a space just for them.

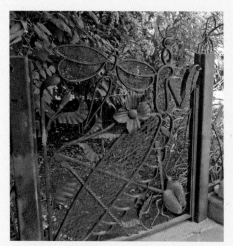

An artful, child-sized gate features a giant metal praying mantis.

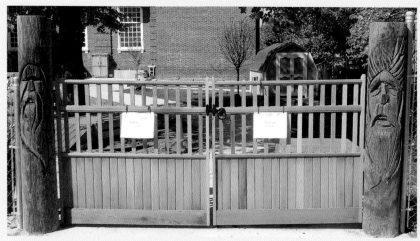

Custom-carved end posts create an intriguing welcome to a schoolyard.

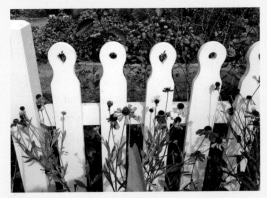

Playful cutout shapes along the top of a simple picket fence gate at the Coastal Maine Botanical Garden announce that fruit is growing nearby.

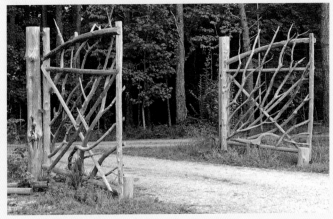

A twigwork entry gate promises a memorable visit.

opportunity to add beauty, sound, invitations to touch something tactile or intriguingly shaped, and perhaps an element of mystery. Above all, the entryway should help the child feel like he or she has arrived *home*—to nature—in the deepest sense.

Entries that take the form of an archway will create the sense of arrival and transitioning from out to in, from there to here. An arbor adds ceremony to the experience. It can be planted with vines that soften the entry and allow one to pass through a wall of greenery. It can also be embellished with moving parts that spin or chime or invite touching. An arch can be small or it can be elongated so that one passes through something like a tunnel to enter the space. There can be one wide arch, or more than one. It is especially respectful to think about scale. Making the entry, or a portion of it, scaled to a child's

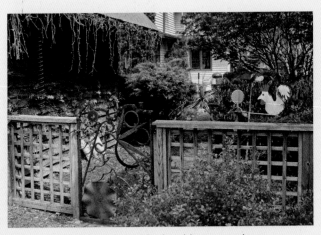

A welcoming garden entry with a hand-hewn metal gate.

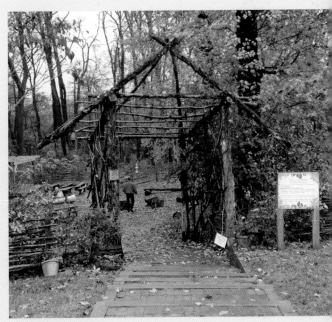

This rustic arbor draws children down the path and into an outdoor classroom.

proportions gives little ones a sense that they were expected and that this place is for them. Having only a child-sized entry that requires adults to crouch down gives children a sense of ownership and says that grownups are guests in the space.

A beautiful gate—perhaps painted a vibrant color, or with added texture or sculptural embellishments—is another way to mark the experience of entering. Chimes, vines, pickets to run a hand or stick along, spinning pinwheels, weather vanes, whirligigs, fluttering flags, and peek-through holes all bring a fanciful element to the space around an entry and will entice children to engage with the space.

It is important to consider the views, the sounds, and the textures underfoot as part of the whole experience of arriving. Whether the view opens to a panorama or disappears temptingly around a curve in the path helps determine how the space will be perceived. Views can entice,

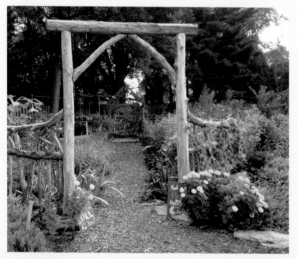

Passing under a beautiful arch creates a clear sense of arrival.

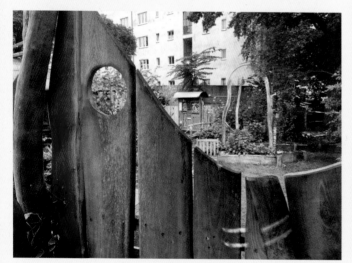

Peepholes can offer a fun perspective on the spaces beyond.

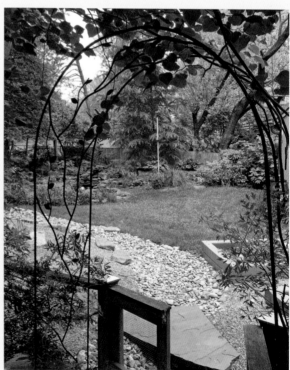

A simple archway with a growing branch motif frames an inviting view into the garden.

reassure, and assuage fears. Youngsters arriving at school or childcare, or any new or busy place, can use a view into the space and the activity there to understand what to expect. Providing a place to pause, perhaps a bench at the entry, allows one to observe, orient oneself, and enter when ready.

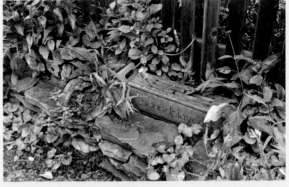

A melodic tongue drum sitting on a low stone wall invites children to stop and play some music.

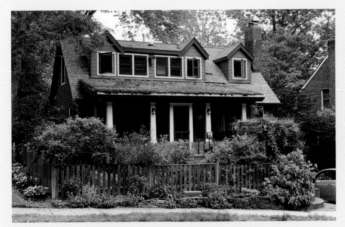

In designing the entry to my own house, I included elements that are welcoming and that provide a clear sense of transition between public and private space.

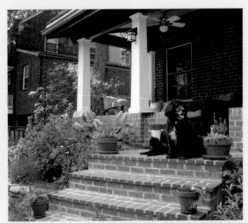

Don't underestimate the role of a welcoming front porch, a sheltered space for family, friends, and pets to gather and overlook life on the block.

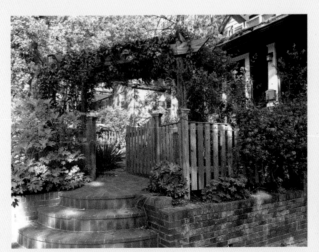

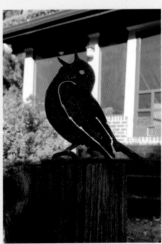

An arbor over a corner entrance to the yard extends the sense of arrival and leads to a little front garden sanctuary laden with flowers, fragrance, and art—such as a metal sculpture of a singing bird—and the sound of a burbling fountain.

The entry to my own garden is designed as a sequence of layers, moving progressively from open and public to sheltered and private. The outer layer, a stone wall against the public sidewalk, is planted with child-friendly lamb's ears, lemon balm, and mint, along with flowers and grasses. These plants welcome strolling children and adults with fragrance, color, texture, and an invitation to pick some herbs. Perched atop the low stone wall is a tongue drum with a sign that says "play," inviting passersby to pause, interact, and send some beautiful sounds wafting through the neighborhood. Up a few steps from the street is my house. One passes through a gate topped with a tiny metal bird sculpture and under an arbor planted with vines to enter the private front garden, which is filled with flowers, fragrance, and the sound of water overflowing a stone bowl fountain into a bed of smooth rocks.

A stepping-stone path leads through the garden and around the house, but the main brick walk leads up a few more steps and onto the porch, a sheltered transition space that connects indoors to out. It is a space where as a family, or

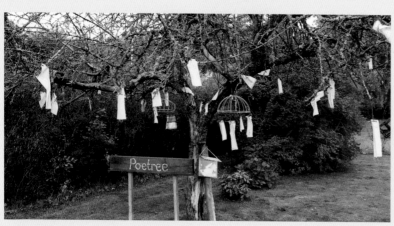

Friendly communities share generously between neighbors. A vegetable bed moved to a front yard not only brings color and life to the street, it invites more interaction than a lawn does.

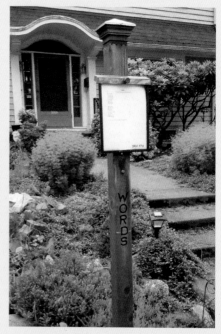

This house isn't for sale. A closer look reveals that the resident poet is sharing work.

A "poetree" invites writers to display their work.

with our friends, we can sit and visit, eat, read, or watch the birds, the rain, or life on the street—all from a protected perch. A carefully conceived entry can bring magic to a whole family's day.

I believe that such invitations demonstrate caring and create a sense of community. Take a cue from the Little Free Library boxes that dot neighborhoods across the country and think about ways to incorporate similar nature-inspired invitations to people walking down your own street. Sharing small moments sends an important message to and about your community. A swing hung from a tree close to the curb, a poem about nature posted near a sidewalk, a fairy house with invitations to arrange and interact: all of these convey a sense of welcome and friendliness, especially when natural materials are used.

More and more schools and parks are creating natural playscapes, and you can adapt things you see in these public spaces for your own home yard or neighborhood pocket park. For example, the entrance to Creative Minds International Public Charter School in Washington, DC, is marked with a covered pergola. Just inside the entry arch is a circular area with two rustic benches that serve as gathering spaces for transitions. This circle provides a site where children can pause, orient, and prepare for what is to come. It also encourages children, teachers, and parents to gather and chat right at the entry. Completing the space is a carved chameleon (the school's mascot), an endearing welcome.

Entry areas can tell arrivals something about who made the space and what it is intended for. At Drew Model Elementary School in Arlington, Virginia, the entry path into its Reading Garden is the Word Walk, a concrete path with language arts terms pressed into the paving. This element is meant to welcome visitors and add texture and interest to the ground beneath their feet, while

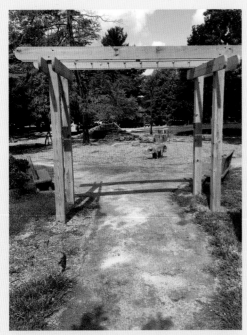

This pergola frames an inviting view into the play space. Right at the entry, children can see that this is definitely a place for them.

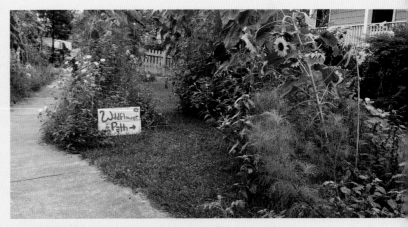

A handmade sign invites passersby to step off the sidewalk to enjoy being enclosed by flowers and greenery.

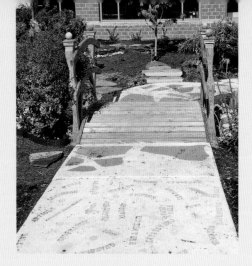

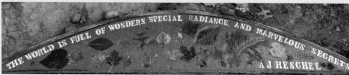

Families can press leaves, names, birthdates, or favorite quotes into concrete to personalize pathways through a yard. Wet concrete is an almost irresistible invitation to children.

presenting curriculum in an unconventional and engaging way. Teachers provided lists of favorite literary terms and the walk became a uniquely physical way for children to connect to the words. You could adapt this at home by pressing a new concrete path with words meaningful to your family, names of family members, or even names of trees and plants in your yard.

PATHS

Circulation refers to the ways people travel through a given space, a key element of how well any space works. Paths—their width and materials, where they lead—tell children a lot about how to move through an outdoor space. Wide-open pathways tell kids that this is a place where they can move quickly and in big, exuberant groups. A narrow stepping-stone path says this is a place to move more slowly and carefully and probably single file. Thoughtful planning can provide important cognitive and motor experiences for children.

The very existence of a path tells us that we are following where others have gone before and there is comfort in that knowledge. Paths can include a view that will draw children along to an engaging play element. Serpentine paths can be mysterious and spur curiosity about what might be around the next bend.

Pathways, stepping stones, bridges, and tunnels transport us on our journeys, adding a sense of adventure. A good path helps us read the space and can clarify the way through. For both large

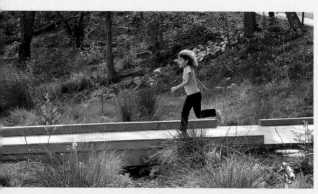

Run free! A long, straight boardwalk through wetlands invites children to move at a gallop.

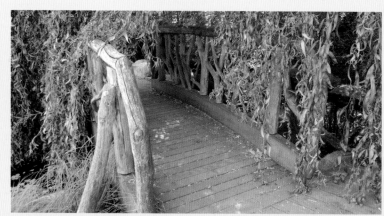

This path disappears intriguingly under a weeping willow.

and small spaces, details in the surfacing, the shape of the path, the terrain, and the landmarks along the way make the route memorable and help us to form mental maps. This in turn allows us to picture the space when we aren't there, describe it to others, and find our way next time. Shortcuts, secondary spurs, and loops can be narrower than the main path and made of different materials. These might lead to unique destinations—a hidden boulder or a special view. Or they

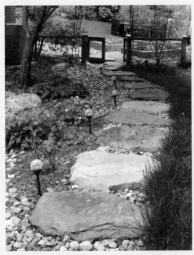

Uneven steps require travelers on the path to pay attention, as the view draws them along.

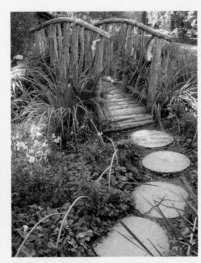

A stepping stone path leads small feet through the garden while also protecting plants.

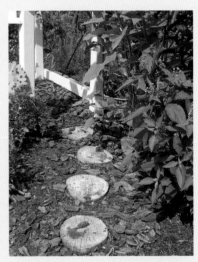

Stepping "stones" made of tree cookies and two contrasting textures of mulch let children get close to plants without trampling them.

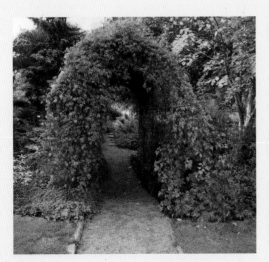

Passing through an enclosed tunnel along a path changes the light, the sound, and the whole experience.

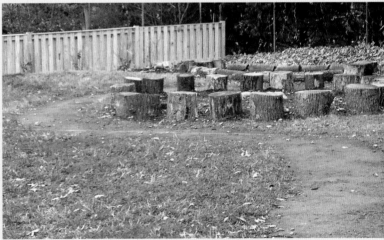

Graceful curves in a gravel path guide children through the space and naturally reduce foot traffic on the lawn.

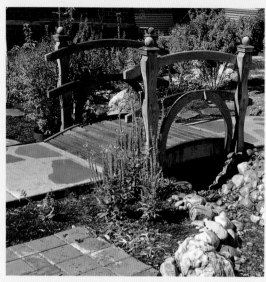

The openness underneath makes walking on a bridge feel and sound hollow—very different from solid ground. Children notice this!

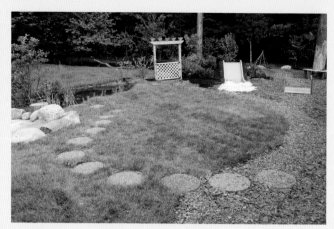

The main path is wood chips, but round stone steps offer a shortcut across the grass, empowering small visitors by giving them a choice of routes.

might just be an interesting side trip off the main path. The opportunity to make choices gives children a sense of control, and offering a selection of routes through the space empowers children. Paths should always lead somewhere, and loops are best for avoiding traffic jams.

It is important to think about the sensory experiences children have as they travel along paths. Surfacing with different textures can change the way pathways are experienced. The crunch of stone dust or pea gravel, the hollow clomp of a boardwalk, the rustle of walking on dry leaves, and the silence of a mulch path all feel and sound very different, deeply affecting our experience of a space. When we are alone or walking quietly, sound can add a meditative quality, helping us to be in the moment and notice each footstep.

Paths can be direct and efficient or meandering and leisurely. Thoughtfully designed walkways can impact behavior in certain parts of the

space and reduce the need for rules or repetitive verbal reminders. A clear path across a flower bed can lead a child through without blossoms being crushed. A route through a rain garden can allow immersion in the space without small feet compacting vulnerable soil. In these ways, paths can safely bring children close to nature without risking harm to what is delicate.

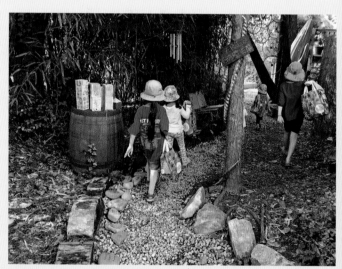

A richly textured, pebbled walkway edged with natural materials and artistic elements draws children along and around a bend.

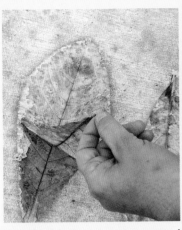
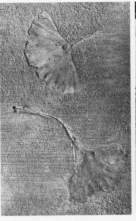
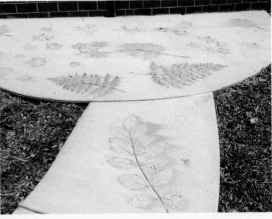

Press fresh leaves into wet concrete. As the concrete cures, the leaves will dry. They can be left to scuff away or can be removed gently. Look for unique and beautiful leaves, such as those of ferns or a ginkgo tree. An assortment of leaves can enhance even the simplest or most utilitarian concrete path.

If you're making paths out of concrete (which is a good way to ensure accessibility for all), remember that this material also provides an opportunity for creativity. Concrete should never be just a smooth (boring) surface. Press plant parts—leaves, ferns, flowers—into the wet mix to make beautiful fossil-like impressions when the concrete dries and the organic matter scuffs away.

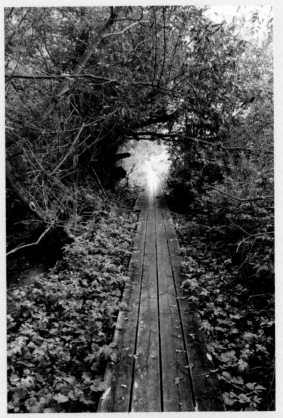

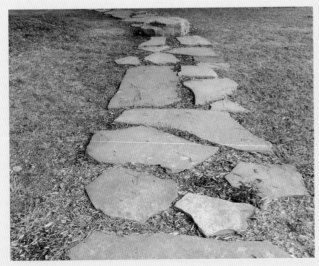

A flagstone walk feels very solid underfoot, and the arrangement of stepping stones gives children choices about which ones to jump, step, or tiptoe on.

A long, straight boardwalk produces a hollow sound. The open, light area ahead will draw kids down the path.

PIZZA BOX PAVER STEPPING STONES

WHAT YOU'LL NEED

* cardboard pizza boxes
* scissors or knife for cutting cardboard
* duct tape
* sheers for cutting hardware cloth
* hardware cloth or chicken wire
* non-stick oil spray such as PAM
* ready-mix concrete in bags (a 40-lb. bag makes approximately six 14-inch squares)
* wheelbarrow or plastic basin
* water source
* sturdy shovel
* lots of fresh (not dry) leaves
* trowel

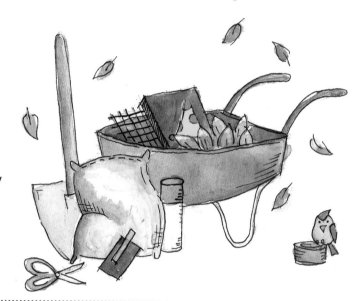

1. Clear a space where the boxes full of wet concrete will be able to dry undisturbed for a day or so.

2. Prep the boxes: cut off the top, reinforce around the edges with duct tape.

3. Cut the hardware cloth or chicken wire into squares just a little smaller than the pizza box. Be careful, it can be sharp.

4. Spray the inside of the pizza box with oil. This will make removing the finished stepping stone much easier.

5. Mix up the concrete according to instructions.

6. Place the pizza box in the spot you've prepared. You won't want to move it once it's full of wet concrete.

7. Set a square of hardware cloth or chicken wire in the box. This helps keep the concrete from cracking later.

8. Scoop wet concrete into the box and smooth it off with a trowel when it is at or just below the top of the box. You want the finished steps to be as thick as possible.

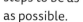

9 Press green leaves into the wet concrete, vein-side down. Vary the designs. One big leaf print can be very dramatic, a pattern made with many leaves can be intricate and interesting. Don't overlap the leaves. Detach leaves from branches, even small ones.

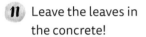

10 Smooth over the leaves with the trowel. Don't worry if some concrete gets on top of the leaves.

11 Leave the leaves in the concrete!

12 When the concrete has set up *completely* (this varies depending on whether the steppers are in the sun and what the air temperature is) and the leaves are dry and brittle, tear off the cardboard and peel off the leaves.

13 Arrange your stepping stones into a path.

14 To make the path more stable, set each stepping stone into the ground. Do this by cutting around each one with a shovel, moving the stone and digging out the soil. Set the stepper back into the cutout hole. You may have to add or scrape away soil to get the stepping stone to sit solidly without rocking.

15 Enjoy your beautiful path!

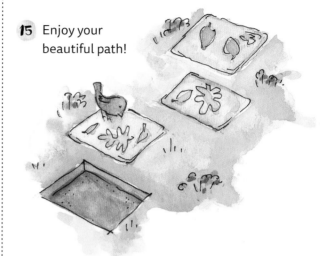

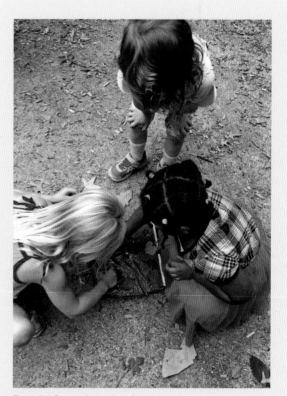

Pressing leaves into pizza box pavers.

Pathways can incorporate a variety of textures that will make walking, running, and riding more interesting and require us to be attentive. Natural stone, whether cut into precise squares and rectangles or broken into irregular shapes, will be long lasting and beautiful. Tree cookies in different diameters can be a ground-level path, or, if varying thicknesses and heights are used, can add a balance challenge to the route.

Children can make stepping stones out of concrete and embellish them with tile, marbles, shells, and stones to add color and texture. Planting scented herbs between steppers allows fragrance to be released as a child walks along the path—adding another sensory dimension to movement through the space. Plants can be neat and obedient with clear edges, or they can spill into the

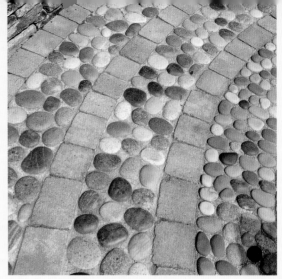

River rock and pavers set in a concrete path designed for barefoot walking create a unique tactile experience.

pathway at different heights, brushing against our legs or creating leafy curtains to push through.

Studies tell us that many of today's children are less physically competent than children of the past. This is happening in other countries as well as the United States. In Germany, recent accident statistics showed increasing numbers of adults were being injured by falls while walking. In Germany, unlike in the United States, insurance is provided by the government, which influences their view of risk and litigation. The

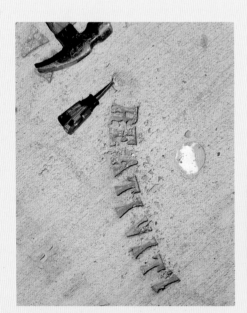

To make the Word Walk at the Drew Model School Reading Garden in Arlington, Virginia, I pressed wooden letters purchased from a craft store into the concrete. When the concrete was dry, I popped the letters out with a screwdriver.

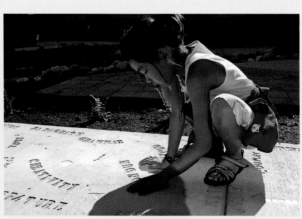

The result is a walkway of imprinted words.

national health insurer approached the agency that designs play spaces and requested that more uneven surfaces be included in children's spaces so that young people would learn to move more attentively, develop better balance, and reduce the number of costly injuries when they reached adulthood! To make your pathways engaging and challenging, think about including a mix of cobblestones, bricks, flat pavers, flagstone, river rocks, tree cookies, and timbers. Even simple treatments to paths can encourage children to move creatively through an outdoor space.

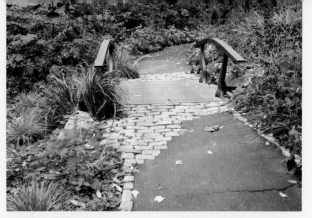

Cobblestones mark a pathway bridge, adding a visual cue and contrast.

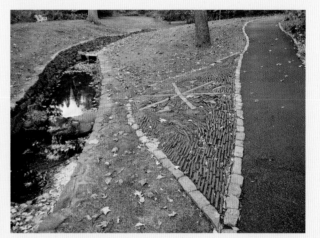

A textured offshoot of a smooth, straight path provides a spot to pause and enjoy the view.

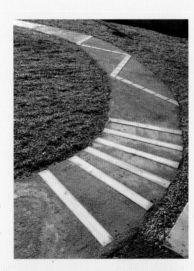

A stone dust path inlaid with wood and bricks provides variety for a child's eyes and feet.

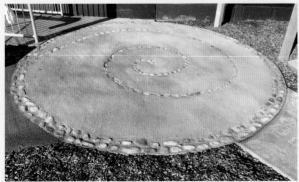

River rocks enhance this concrete circle and encourage following the spiral path.

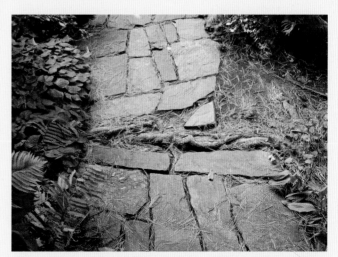

An arrangement of irregular pavers incorporates tree roots into the path, protecting the tree, celebrating and exposing its root system, and making the path more interesting.

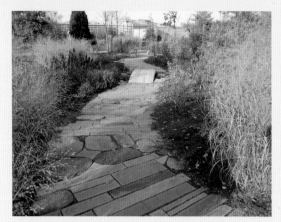

Soft grasses, meandering curves and undulations, and a mix of pavers engage multiple senses.

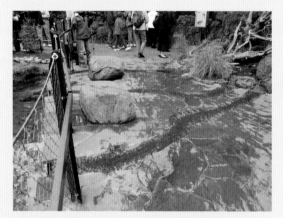

Little stone rills set into paving allow water to flow across a path, inviting splashing and touching.

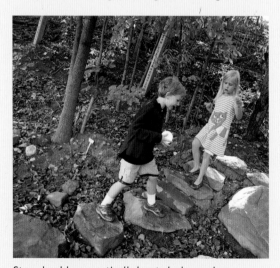

Stone boulders practically beg to be hopped on.

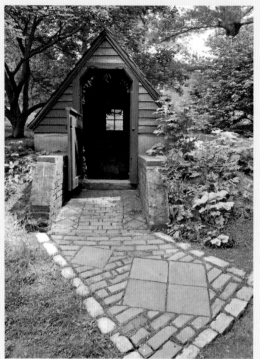

Pavers don't have to be straight or perfect. Askew is more interesting—especially to children.

FRIENDLY FENCING

The elements that children encounter as they travel along a path, or that help keep them safely confined in a space, can be thoughtfully designed to add richness and to underscore a use of natural materials. Think about how the boundaries around a space might vary in height and openness and texture, and what that will convey to a child. Simple rope or rail, lattice or screen, solid low logs, or solid full shrubs can give kids something to crouch behind or peer over. Handrails along a path can vary in height and materials: consider wood, metal pipes, chains, ropes. Pickets and fence infill can be made of different materials as well, such as wood, metal, mirrors, glass, wire, and woven mats, each with different degrees of openness or transparency.

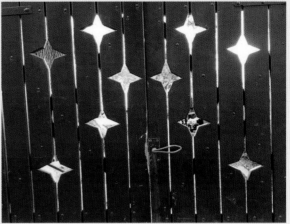

Cut patterns provide glimpses into the space beyond and also let slivers of light through.

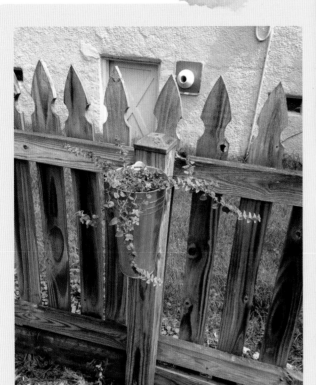

Plants hung in a galvanized metal pail soften a fence.

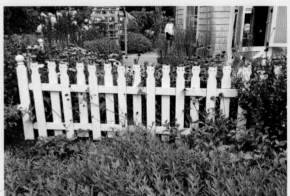

Kitty cat pickets transform a fence into a playful sculpture at the Coastal Maine Botanical Gardens.

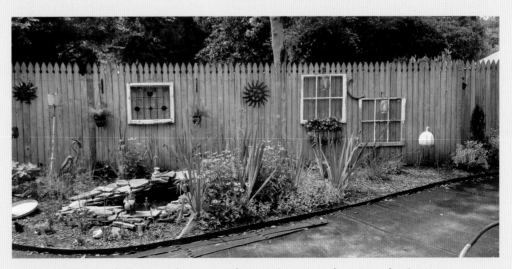

An artful collection of old window frames transforms a plain privacy fence into a focal point.

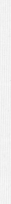

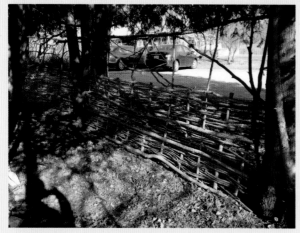

Saplings woven between trees form a solid lower fence without obscuring the view for taller folks.

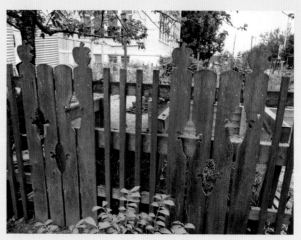

Fancifully shaped cutouts in pickets give a classic American fence personality.

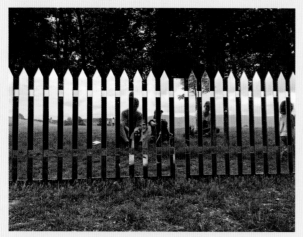

For high drama, consider pickets made of acrylic mirror to bring the reflected sky views and light down into the landscape, as artist Alyson Shotz created at the Storm King Art Center in upstate New York.

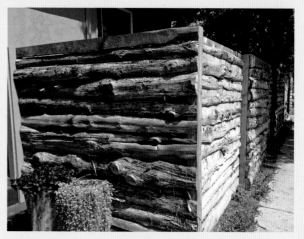

A solid privacy fence that exposes the bark and uneven knots of logs creates a rough and interesting surface, as well as a clearly defined edge to the space it encloses.

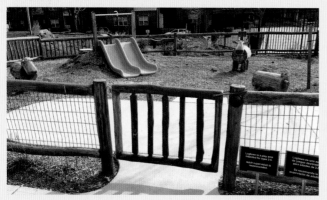

An open wire grid framed with locust logs creates a safe enclosure with an open feel.

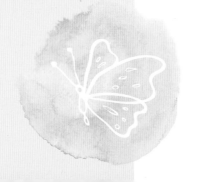

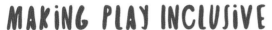

MAKING PLAY INCLUSIVE

Always be mindful of accessibility for children and others who use mobility assistance devices when creating the main pathway through a space. The route can be interesting and varied, and it should not be prohibitively uneven. Secondary paths can be narrower and include things such as irregular stepping stones.

All-terrain wheels or wheelchairs may be an option for some. When a pathway is challenging (because of a crack, slick spot, or intentional design component) or impossible for some to use, consider a different paradigm. Encourage children, with and without mobility challenges, to work together to include everyone. The reality is that the whole world will probably never be completely accessible, so it is important for all children to feel comfortable and empowered to offer *and* to ask for help when needed. The outdoors provides opportunities for empathy and understanding to grow in children.

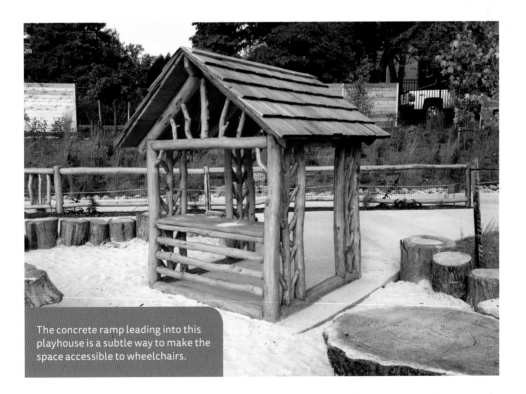

The concrete ramp leading into this playhouse is a subtle way to make the space accessible to wheelchairs.

Pathway Plants for Color, Texture, and Fragrance

Dwarf chamomile* (*Chamaemelum nobile* 'Treneague') A non-flowering, miniature chamomile with fragrant leaves.

Miniature moneywort* (*Lysimachia japonica* var. *minutissima*) A tiny-leafed plant that forms a dense mat between steps. Yellow flowers.

Mint* (*Mentha*) Peppermint, spearmint, lemon mint, curly mint, Corsican mint—plant any of these alongside a path to add texture and fragrance when crushed or brushed. Make sure mint is contained by pots or edges, however, so it doesn't take over! Snip a leaf to chew on or to flavor your lemonade.

Oregano* (*Origanum vulgare* 'Humile') A low-growing, fragrant herb that is also delicious on your pizza or in spaghetti sauce.

Thyme* (*Thymus*) There are many varieties of thyme that creep and fill in between stepping stones, adding color, texture, and delicious fragrance when crushed underfoot. Also yummy in chicken soup. Woolly thyme (*Thymus pseudolanuginosus*) is an extra-soft species that feels great underfoot.

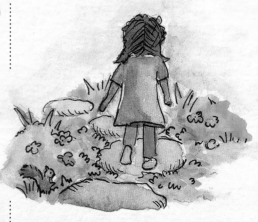

Woolly yarrow* (*Achillea tomentosa*) Yellow flowers, soft, low-growing, creeping foliage.

* Indicates non-native North American plants.

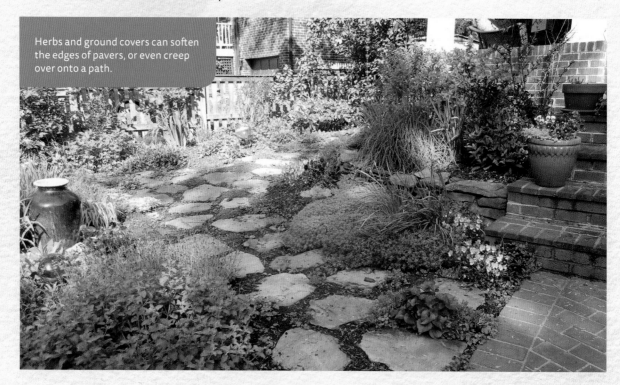

Herbs and ground covers can soften the edges of pavers, or even creep over onto a path.

NICHES, NOOKS, AND OUTDOOR ROOMS

Places to pause, like benches or defined alcoves, create interest along the way to a destination. We can think about organizing the outdoors similarly to the way we think about interior spaces. In a house, each room has its own feeling—the kitchen has a different purpose than the living room, and looks and feels different in order to support what goes on there. This can happen outside as well. There can be a variety of "rooms," each with its own energy, mood, purpose, and capacity. The degree of openness or enclosure is one way to define these areas; another is with the materials we use above, below, and around the space. Some areas might need to be defined and enclosed, others might offer a view out. The size of outdoor rooms should vary as well, with some large enough for a group to gather, others for pairs to play, and some private places just big enough for one.

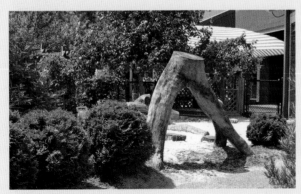

This inviting space at the Otto Wels School in Berlin, Germany, has garden beds, artful trellises, and a comfy pair of seats around a lush lawn.

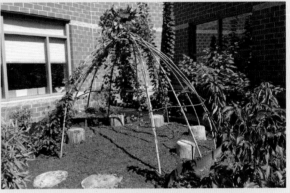

Places to pause along the way: a simple bamboo-pole bower encloses a circle of stump seats. As the vines grow up the poles, the interior will become increasingly shady and enclosed.

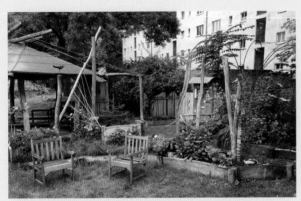

The crotch of a tree destined to be cut down was carefully harvested, flipped, and braced to create a memorable entry to a sandpit.

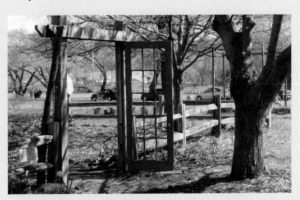

A doorway, the taken-for-granted entrance within a structure, becomes a fun outdoor surprise.

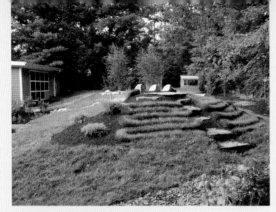

Compost logs planted with grass enclose an entry path leading up to a small platform. These fabric tubes filled with compost absorb rainwater like a sponge and help prevent erosion on a hillside. They don't like a lot of foot traffic, though.

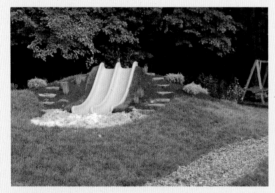

This low hill was sculpted into the space to add a different vantage point and room for a short slide.

Niches and nooks needn't be sequestered from view to be meaningful or distinct. Take advantage of your terrain's natural topographical features or sculpt it to create special spots: elevated vantage points like hills and berms; low spaces like gullies, swales, and hollows; wide open lawns and fields; and protected caves and tunnels carved out of a slope. Areas with inclines, terraces, and undulating paths—not to mention colorful, fragrant, or textural plants—all make an area more captivating to children and help them orient in the space.

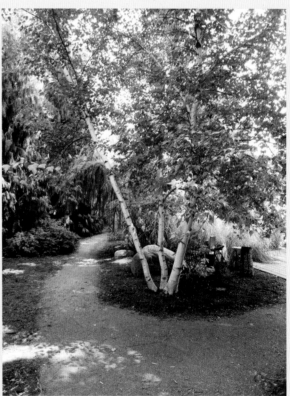

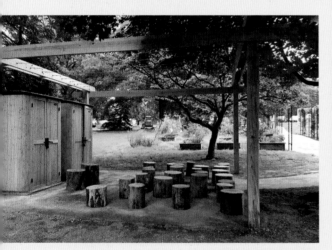

A change in surfacing and an open-frame pergola with wire infill makes it clear where this garden classroom begins and ends. Scale this for your backyard by creating a smaller pergola and providing seats for family members and friends.

A rest stop along a path is a place to pause, with a sitting rock in the shade of a clump of birches.

The height and materials of an outdoor room's "ceiling" can vary, from soft plant canopies to rocky cave overhangs, airy trellises to low tunnel roofs. Overhead enclosures can be solid or have openings to let light through, and light levels may vary. The leafy branches of a tree define the height and openness of the space below, in the way the limbs drape or curve.

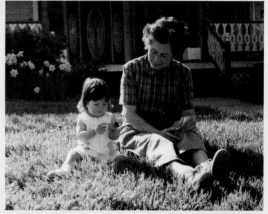

A bit of lawn is the perfect place for baby (my daughter, many years ago) and her grandmother to sit together.

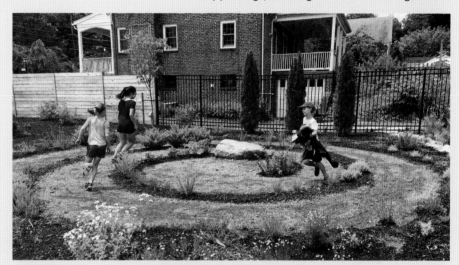

A labyrinth or spiral path can encourage meditative walks or fast and silly chases.

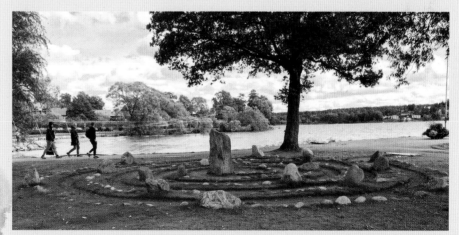

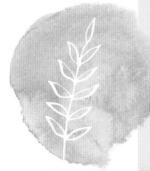

Large stones give a monolithic feel to a circular lakeside walk in Altuna, Sweden.

Varied surfacing on the ground throughout the space can help create different moods. Decks and patios are obvious examples of spaces defined by the surfacing. No material is without its pros and cons, so employ a variety if you have the room: cool grass for sitting and running; sand, soft mulch, and perhaps wood chips for easy landings; gravel for good drainage and crunch underfoot; decking, stone, pavers, concrete, or asphalt for sturdiness and definition.

Furnishings are another component of outdoor rooms. These could include seating, tables, work surfaces, storage, or the play elements you decide to incorporate.

The purpose of the space should help determine what goes into, above, below, and around it. A colorful and busy art area, a quiet zone for reading, an open place for active play, a spot for cooking and eating, or a performance space: each area should include all the necessary elements to make it functional and comfortable for children and the adults who may be with them.

PUTTING IT ALL TOGETHER

There are many ways to organize a collection of outdoor rooms. For example, in a typical backyard, you may want to leave open space in the center with interesting elements or zones arranged around the edges, allowing visual access across the space. An area can also be arranged as a series of open and enclosed spaces and niches unfolding along a main path. You may have space for only a few outdoor rooms or many.

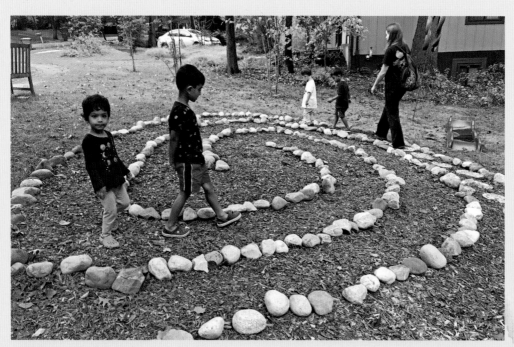

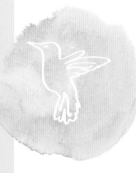

River rock spirals built by children can help teach mindfulness as kids learn to walk slowly and meditatively.

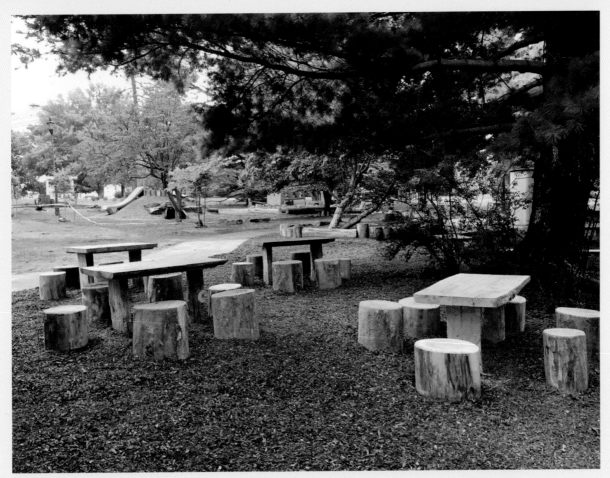

At home, a picnic table in the shade next to the vegetable garden would connect gardening with eating, as this communal arrangement suggests.

Group related elements together: an outdoor cooking and dining area might include a pizza oven, a vegetable garden, a shaded picnic table, and a water source. A building area would need loose parts and a place to store them, skeleton structures, and open space on the ground for building. A place for sensory play could have a lot of sand, perhaps a water source, work surfaces, shade, and places to sit. A performance space might contain a simple stage, musical instruments, seating for an audience, and storage for costumes and props.

Views from different perspectives help children understand the space, a skill known as mental mapping. Think about taking advantage of scenes along a pathway or from an overlook, enhancing surprise views as you round a corner, framing a panoramic sight with plantings, or creating peek holes and port holes into spaces beyond.

Dedicate space to outdoor areas for activities you or your children love, such as a rustic outdoor dining table for backyard meals.

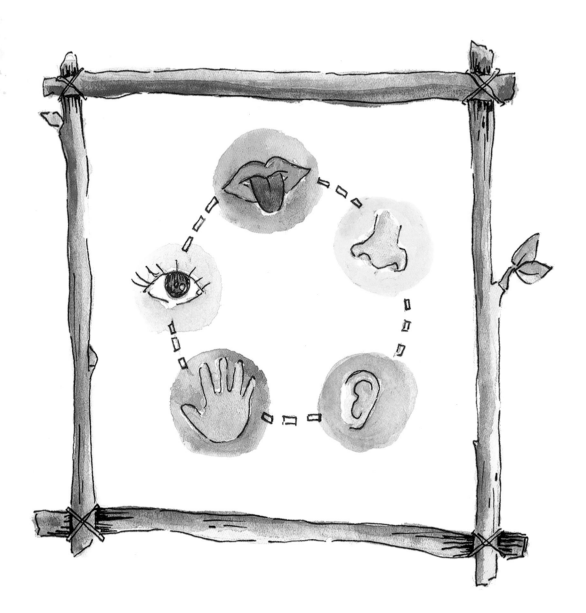

Awakening Senses

"Being outdoors can provide
a sense of freedom."

—from *The Great Outdoors*, by Mary Rivkin

Nature nourishes all our senses. From the sweet scent of fragrant flowers and the whisper of breezes through tall grass, to the arresting beauty of foliage colors and the taste of juicy, sun-warmed berries. Even the feel of the earth itself awakens perception: warm stone, cool water, crumbly dirt, sticky mud. Nature can bring fascinating, soothing, richly engaging sensory experiences to children's lives.

For young brains, interacting and experimenting with these essential elements provides a direct connection to the most powerful pathways for knowing: hands-on, deep engagement. Children learn through all their senses. Immersion in the smells, sounds, sights, textures, tastes, and temperatures of nature forms a foundation for understanding the physical realm, for creativity, and for a sense of ourselves as part of a bigger world.

Humans need consistency and some measure of predictability to feel secure, but variety and change are crucial to being engaged with the world. Nature is the perfect source of this subtle equilibrium between difference and sameness. The echo of a burbling stream as water flows over uneven pebbles, the whisper of leaves blowing in a gentle breeze, the dance of flames in a bonfire—each offers the balance of consistency and gentle surprise our senses crave.

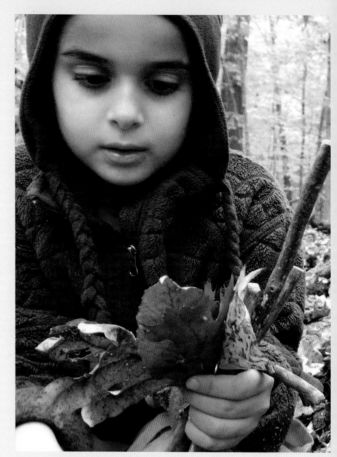

Fallen autumn leaves offer a rich variety of sensory input, including colors, textures, and crunching underfoot.

SENSORY LEARNING

In this chapter we will explore the five senses: smell, hearing, touch, sight, and taste—plus two more from the world of sensorimotor integration: the proprioceptive sense and the vestibular sense. When children use their muscles and the force of their bodies to push or dig or roll or lift heavy things, they become aware of their own bodies' capabilities and develop a sense of where they are in space. This is the proprioceptive sense. The vestibular sense relates to our sense of balance. Sensory processing disorder (SPD) refers to children who are more, or less, sensitive to sensory stimulation than the average. For all children, but especially those with SPD, unstructured time soaking up nature at their own pace through their senses can be very therapeutic, especially when combined with support that helps children develop empathy, awareness, and mindfulness.

Smell

If you think back to your own childhood, scent is probably something that triggers powerful memories. The aroma of lilacs in spring always takes me back to the grove where I played when I was young. Think about the smell of a forest after rain, a salt marsh at low tide, or animals on a farm. In each case, the scent forms a powerful aspect of the identity of that space in our minds.

As you work to create memorable play spaces for your own children, consider that potency and try to incorporate plants whose blooms have distinctive, pleasing scents: place gardenia and viburnum at key spots along pathways, jasmine near the front door, and lilacs outside of bedroom windows to waft in on summer nights.

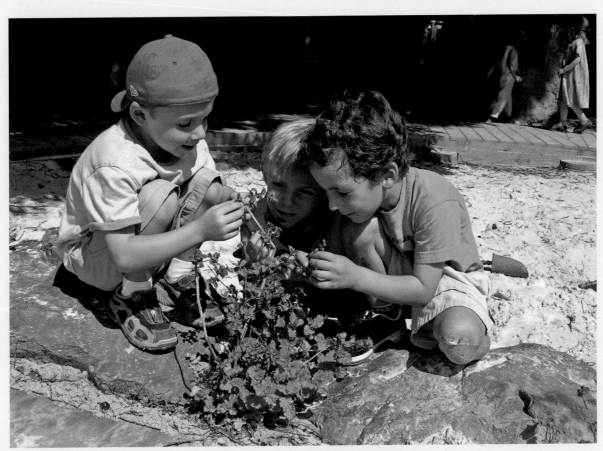

Pickable and aromatic mint is planted between boulders that separate a path from a sandpit.

PLANTS for SMELLING

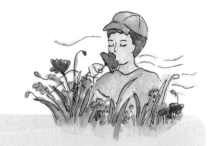

PLANT	DESCRIPTION
PERENNIAL HERBS	
Chives* (*Allium schoenoprasum*)	Pretty (and edible) purple flowers in spring. The stalks of this onion-scented plant are fun to chew before kissing Mom with onion breath (also great stir-fried or added to salad).
Lemon balm* (*Melissa officinalis*)	Lemon balm has square stems, so it is in the mint family, but its powerful lemony fragrance has not a hint of the scent of mint. Good for tea, or just rub or chew on the leaf to release a powerful scent.
Mint* (*Mentha* species)	Plants in the mint family can be identified by their square stems. They are generally aggressive growers, which can be controlled by planting in containers, or, in my experience, by the little feet that tend to tromp over them when planted in a play space. Includes American mint, peppermint*, spearmint*, chocolate mint*, pineapple mint*, orange mint*, curly mint* and many more. Explore your local garden center to find the scents you like best. Delicious in tea, coated with chocolate, or ground for homemade toothpaste.
Mountain mint (*Pycnanthemum virginianum*)	A fragrant native that brings scent when brushed up against or crushed. The late summer and autumn blossoms are a pollinator magnet.
Rosemary* (*Rosmarinus officinalis*)	Part of a large family of evergreen herbs native to dry Mediterranean climates. Yummy roasted with potatoes or added to a rub on pork or lamb. Just rub the leaves and release the fragrance. In Shakespeare's time it was said that rosemary helped with memory, so a sprig behind the ear ought to help to ace the next test at school.
Thyme* (*Thymus vulgaris*)	A semievergreen, low-growing woody herb. Nice planted among stepping stones, where it releases its distinct fragrance when stepped on. Often used in cooking. Try it in chicken soup or scrambled eggs.
FRAGRANT FLOWERS AND FOLIAGE	
Hay-scented fern (*Dennstaedtia punctilobula*)	This fern loves dry shade and turns soft yellow in the fall. When crushed, the foliage smells just as the name implies.
Hyacinth* (*Hyacinthus* species)	Plant bulbs in the fall for knock-your-socks-off fragrant blooms in the early spring. The flowers, leaves, and stems completely disappear by summer.
Woodland phlox (*Phlox divaricata*)	Sweet-smelling blue flowers appear in late winter or early spring. Perfect in a partly shady spot, such as a woodland fairy garden.

PLANT	DESCRIPTION
FRAGRANT WOODY SHRUBS	
Fall-blooming witch hazel (*Hamamelis virginiana*)	Twisty, sweet-scented flowers bloom in fall, but can sometimes be hidden by the great fall leaf color.
Fothergilla (*Fothergilla* species)	Fragrant honey-puff flowers appear in early spring; gorgeous orangey leaf color delights in fall.
Gardenia* (*Gardenia* species)	Gardenias likes sunny but protected areas. Look for blooms throughout summer. This evergreen shrub isn't hardy everywhere, but if you can grow it, you should, because the scent is heavenly. You'll never forget it and when you smell it, the memory will whisk you back to wherever you were when you first breathed it in.
Koreanspice viburnum* (*Viburnum carlesii*)	Pinkish white blooms are deliciously fragrant in early to midspring.
Lilac* (*Syringa* species)	Late-spring blooms in lavender and white have an unforgettably beautiful scent.
Native azalea (*Rhododendron* species)	This shrub has lots of colors and bloom times (varieties include coast azalea, swamp azalea, flame azalea, and pinxterbloom azalea). All attract hummingbirds and most are extremely fragrant, unlike the evergreen variety from Asia.
Spicebush (*Lindera benzoin*)	This plant likes wet, sunny, or shady spots. Leaves are fragrant when crushed.
Spring-blooming witch hazel (*Hamamelis vernalis*)	Twisty, sweet-scented flowers bloom in early spring. Yellow and orange foliage is an autumn highlight.
Summersweet (*Clethra alnifolia*)	Lightly fragrant, soft pink or white flowers appear in summer.
Sweet bay magnolia (*Magnolia virginiana*)	A semievergreen tree with waxy, white, lemon-scented flowers in spring. Grows best in moist soil.
Sweet box* (*Sarcococca hookeriana* var. *humilis*)	Late winter and early spring blooms. Flowers on this small evergreen are tiny and difficult to see, but the scent is impossible to miss. Great planted near the front door or along any path you'll be using when these flowers are in bloom.

*Indicates non-native. All other plants listed are North American natives.

Hearing

Listening for and locating sounds in nature help children understand that space is three-dimensional: birds call from high in the trees, the humming of insects can come from deep in the weeds. And whether it's rustling grasses or chimes overhead, the sounds of nature can soothe us. Consider including elements that will purposefully add a variety of sounds.

We often ask children to use their "indoor" voices, so once outdoors, kids should have opportunities to explore different levels of sound and music-making. Yelling, howling, and singing at the top of one's lungs, as well as making sounds with drums and other instruments are all ways the outdoors can give children opportunities to experiment and develop (literally) their own voices. Whether we use manufactured instruments or things we make—tubes to blow in, whisper phones, things to tap and drum on such as buckets, pots, pans, pipes, pickets, and wood slats—big, loud, exuberant noise is often best created outside.

SOUND STATIONS

You can enhance an arbor or trellis in your space by hanging chimes, bells, or percussion instruments from the structure. If you don't have such a frame, you can also use a pair of posts to support a pipe or a beam, then screw hooks into the beam and hang a changing array of percussion pieces: metal pots and pans; plastic trash cans and buckets of all sizes; and hollow pipes made of bamboo, PVC, or metal in different diameters and lengths. You can also add things like wood pickets, wagon or bicycle wheels, xylophones, drums, and natural materials like sea shells. Once you begin experimenting with the sounds of different objects, you'll discover that sound stations have infinite potential.

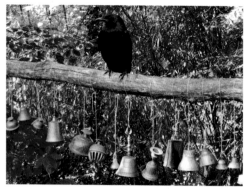

Sally Crow visits a collection of bells suspended from a branch.

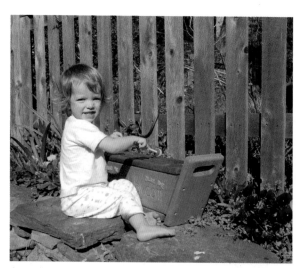

Consider setting some instruments out where neighborhood children can all enjoy them, such as this tongue drum set on a low wall along a public sidewalk.

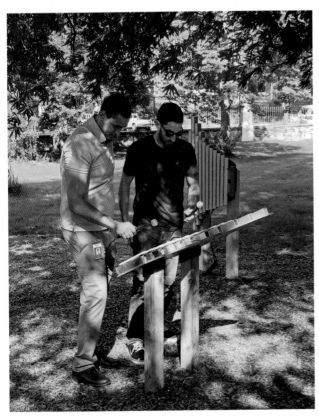

Music teachers discover pentatonic instruments at the opening of a play space.

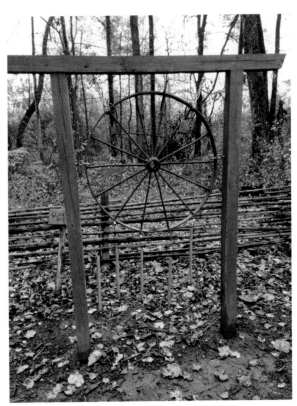

Start looking at found objects with an eye toward their sound-making potential, such as this old wagon wheel mounted on a simple frame.

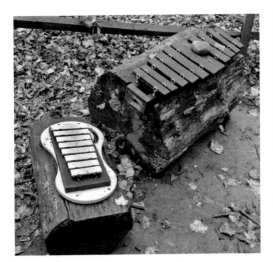

Xylophones embedded in logs recycle indoor instruments and add sturdiness.

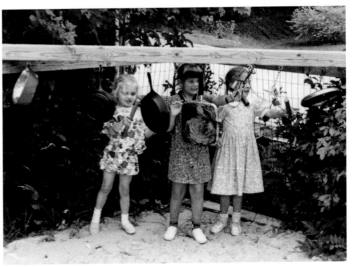

Old pots and pans can have a second life as low-cost musical instruments.

PLANTS for HEARING

PLANT	DESCRIPTION
RUSTLING GRASSES	
River oats (*Chasmanthium latifolium*)	This ornamental grass makes a lovely rustling sound in the breeze. Dense roots make it also good for holding banks and preventing erosion. (However, they can be difficult to get rid of, so plant carefully.)
Prairie dropseed (*Sporobolus heterolepis*)	Native to the American prairie, this fine textured grass grows to about 18 inches tall and turns a lovely golden in autum.
Switch grass (*Panicum virgatum*)	Fluffy, airy panicles float like a cloud above this clumping grass.
RATTLING SEED PODS	
False indigo (*Baptisia australis*)	Perennial with blue flowers in spring. It thrives in shade and produces pods that make noise when dry.
Columbine (*Aquilegia* species)	Perennial with varieties native to almost every part of the U.S. Tiny seeds sit in open cups and are fun to shake and scatter.
Wood poppy (*Stylophorum diphyllum*)	Perennial that thrives in shade, and will seed about, even growing happily in sun. Yellow flowers from spring through late summer. The plant is slightly toxic so don't plant around young children who might taste it. The stems have a striking bright yellow sap that stains.
Redbud (*Cercis canadensis*)	Edible purple spring flowers give way to seed pods that are fun to collect and shake.
Catalpa (*Catalpa* species)	Native tree with beautiful bell-shaped, white-with-purple spotted flowers in spring and foot-long seed pods in fall that turn brown, fall off, and are a pain to clean up or fun to collect, depending on your perspective.
Kentucky coffeetree (*Gymnocladus dioicus*)	Trees come in male and female. The female has showier, fragrant yellow flowers, then produces 10- to 12-inch seed pods which stay on through winter. Native people ate roasted seeds and ground them to make a coffee-like drink. Seeds are toxic before roasting, so never eat them raw.

All plants listed are North American natives.

Touch

Our skin is the largest organ of our bodies, making touch a vital source of stimulation. Tactile engagement is often neglected in creating spaces for children, but it is crucial, especially for babies, young children, and children of all ages with special needs. Opportunities to touch apply to the whole body: hands *and* bare feet need to experience different textures: rough, smooth, soft, hard, hot, and cold. The brush of a gentle breeze, the warmth radiating from a bonfire, bracing winter air.

Nature is rich in texture and tactile variety. The bark on trees and shrubs can be rough, smooth, bumpy, thorny, chunky, peely, blocky. Leaves can be sticky, fuzzy, smooth, prickly, thick, delicate, veiny. Stone can be smooth, round, jagged, hard, crumbly, warm, cold. In contrast, think about what some manufactured playgrounds feature: fiberglass trees and manufactured boulders. Certainly durable and perhaps low maintenance, but what do they teach children about trees and rocks in nature? The best spaces are filled with *real* objects that invite children to touch and poke, to brush up against, to pick and experience.

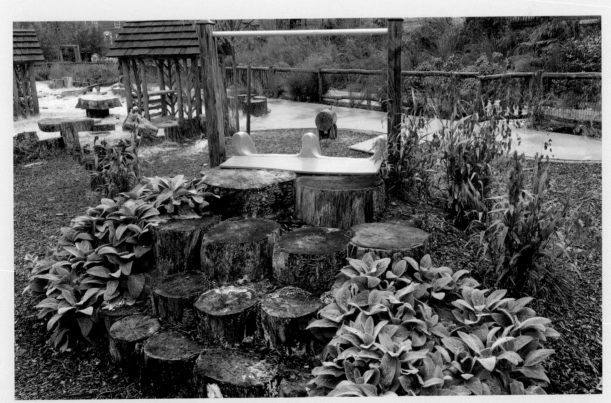

Soft lamb's ears planted alongside a stump scramble offers a tactile treat.

PLANTS for TOUCHING

PLANT	DESCRIPTION
BARK	
American beech (*Fagus grandifolia*)	Soft gray bark that is perfectly smooth.
River birch (*Betula nigra*)	Bark is peely, brown and tan, paperlike sheets that curl and bend.
Red twig dogwood (*Cornus sericea*)	Smooth, glossy, bright red bark.
Musclewood (*Carpinus caroliniana*)	Smooth and ridged bark with definition that makes the trunk look it has like well-developed muscles.
Persimmon (*Diospyros virginiana*)	Grow this tree for the fruit and enjoy the uniquely textured, blocky bark that looks like alligator hide.
Dogwood (*Cornus florida*)	Chunky bark similar to persimmon.
FOLIAGE	
Corkscrew rush (*Juncus effusus* 'Spiralis')	Perennial with a clump of curly, spiraling stems. Thrives in moist to wet soil.
Bluestar (*Amsonia tabernaemontana*)	Soft and feathery foliage is green in summer and warm golden in fall.
Lamb's ears* (*Stachys byzantina*)	Fuzzy leaves really are just like a lamb's ear.
Mexican feather grass (*Nassella tenuissima*)	Wispy, flowy grass that is soft as fur.
Pennsylvania sedge (*Carex pensylvanica*)	Gently arching, soft, grasslike plant for shade. Somewhat delicate but sometimes used for soft lawns in shady yards.
Purple love grass (*Eragrostis spectabilis*)	Thrives in full sun and sandy soil with soft, billowy, reddish purple efflorescence. Grows to 1 to 2 feet tall.
Switch grass (*Panicum virgatum*)	Fluffy, airy panicles float like a cloud above this clumping grass; 2 to 3 feet tall.

*Indicates non-native. All other plants listed are North American natives.

Sight

In a 2013 article published in Slate, Brian Palmer described recent studies in which children who spent time outside in nature were less likely to suffer from myopia (nearsightedness) than their peers who spent more time looking at screens. It makes sense—from examining tiny bugs up close to gazing up at a hawk circling overhead, nature calls on us to look carefully and to focus at different distances. It is important to exercise each and every one of our senses. Having interesting things to look at is paramount, especially for infants and children whose special needs may limit their mobility.

To add visually stimulating motion and color, consider fabric elements such as banners, parachutes, and flags that flap and billow. Whirligigs, mobiles, and weather vanes bring playful movement to the space. Hang prisms in trees to cast magical rainbows around the yard, or glue two CDs together, iridescent sides out, to create the same effect. Provide magnifying glasses for close-up examinations of bugs and leaves, binoculars to bring faraway things close, and kaleidoscopes and fish-eye lenses to fuel a sense of wonder. Just having tall trees with high leaves is a fundamental benefit of being in nature. Big views of the sky—a starry night, thunderclouds, sunsets, sweeping vistas—inspire awe and reverie and are, research tells us, important experiences for a child's developing sense of spirituality and for establishing empathy.

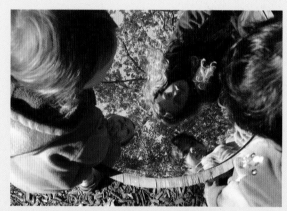

A mirror in the garden creates a striking visual transformation—here it reflects up into the branches and sky.

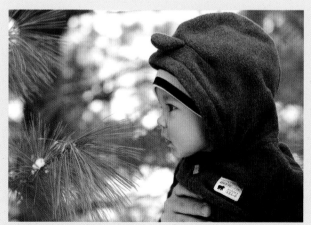

Before babies are even mobile, time outside provides important visual stimulation. Here, during a winter walk, snow-covered pine boughs swaying in the breeze are fascinating.

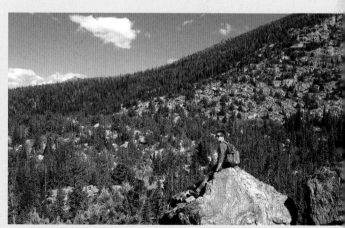

Panoramic views inspire a sense of awe that feeds the soul. In your own backyard, incorporate elements that encourage children to look up, out, and beyond the confines of a fence or hedge.

PLANTS for SEEING

PLANT	DESCRIPTION
REDS, MAGENTAS, PINKS	
Obedient plant (*Physostegia virginiana*)	Perennial offering prolific late-summer and early-fall flowers.
Rose mallow (*Hibiscus moscheutos*)	This perennial produces giant flowers the size of dinner plates in mid- to late summer.
Rose turtlehead (*Chelone obliqua*)	Perennial that blooms in midsummer spikes.
Zinnia* (*Zinnia* species)	A favorite garden annual. Bright, splashy, medium-sized flowers.
ORANGES AND YELLOWS	
Marigold* (*Tagetes* and *Calendula* species)	Annual with selections in a wide range of sizes, all producing yellow to bronze, globe-like flowers throughout summer.
Oxeye daisy (*Heliopsis helianthoides*)	Bright yellow flowers in summer on plants that are 3 to 4 feet tall.
Swamp sunflower (*Helianthus angustifolius*)	Loves wet soil; the plants can be 6 feet tall with an abundance of daisy-like, 2- to 3-inch yellow blooms that last until frost.
Tickseed (*Coreopsis* species)	Features an abundance of mid- to late-summer daisy-like flowers that are great for picking.
BLUES AND PURPLES	
Aster (*Aster* species)	A wide variety of plants with tiny daisy-like flowers from pink to blue to purple, different sizes. All bloom in late summer to frost.
False indigo (*Baptisia australis*)	Striking periwinkle-colored flowers in spring on full, bushy plants that are 3 to 4 feet tall.
Ironweed (*Vernonia noveboracensis*)	Summer to fall blooms, magenta to purple, on plants that are typically 6 to 8 feet tall, depending on variety. 'Iron Butterfly' is only 2 to 3 feet tall. Loves wet soil; good for raingarden.
Morning glory* (various genera)	A climbing vine that produces 4- to 5-inch, sky-blue flowers that only open in the morning.

PLANT	DESCRIPTION
Prairie gay feather (*Liatris spicata*)	Spikey purple flower clusters grow to 2 to 3 feet tall in full sun in early to midsummer.

SPRING COLOR IN A SHADE GARDEN

PLANT	DESCRIPTION
Blue star grass (*Sisyrinchium angustifolium*)	Delicate blue or purple flowers in spring with grasslike foliage. This plant will spread and colonize in sun to part sun.
Columbine (*Aquilegia* species)	Red, orange, or blue spring flowers on various species of this native that grows in shade to part sun and seeds freely around the woodland garden.
Coral bells (*Heuchera americana*)	Look for tiny pink flowers on a tall stem in the spring. Most dramatic feature is foliage—a range of interesting patterns in green, silver, purple, orange, and chartreuse.
Crested iris (*Iris cristata*)	Blue or purple flowers in spring. The 4- to 6-inch-tall foliage spreads to be a nice woodland ground cover.
Green and gold (*Chrysogonum virginianum*)	Brilliant yellow flowers on a low-growing plant that likes to creep and spread in full sun.
Groundsel (*Senecio vulgaris*)	Creeper with yellow flowers. Lovely planted between stepping stones in full sun.
Jack-in-the-pulpit (*Arisaema triphyllum*)	Blue or purple spring flowers on a woodland plant.

STRIKING FALL COLOR

PLANT	DESCRIPTION
American beautyberry (*Callicarpa americana*)	This shrub has tiny white flowers which produce gorgeous magenta berries in autumn. Likes shade to part sun. Yellow in fall. Grows to 6 feet tall.
Fothergilla (*Fothergilla* species)	Flaming orange, purple, and yellow fall leaves. White, fragrant, honey-puff flowers in spring. Shrub that likes sun to part sun and grows to 3 to 9 feet depending on variety.
Hearts-a-Bustin' (*Euonymus americanus*)	A native shrub that grows in the woods. Features one-of-a-kind orange and pink seed pods in fall.
Sumac (*Rhus aromatica, R. typhina* or *R. copallinum*)	A large shrub or small tree that grows in full sun to part sun with brilliant red autumn foliage.

*Indicates non-native. All other plants listed are North American natives.

Taste

It's a special joy to forage and eat wild-growing edibles. Learning to recognize wild foods can begin with a feast of wild mulberries or blackberries, as likely to be found in a city park or alley as along a trail. Kids can learn to recognize salad makings such as young dandelion greens, garlic mustard, wood sorrel, and violet flowers in their own lawns in early spring. (A little dirt builds the immune system, but it's generally a good idea to wash what you forage before you eat, and of course avoid foraging in places where pesticides and herbicides have been sprayed!)

Helping children grow edibles from seeds or seedlings is another way to connect taste with nature, and more important, to the essential dietary role plant foods play in keeping us healthy. I'll speak more to the importance of children growing vegetables and fruit a little later.

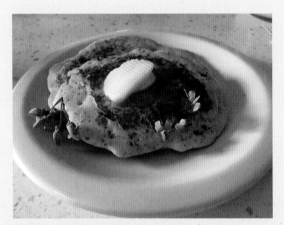

Edible redbud flowers (*Cercis canadensis*) make a weekend breakfast truly memorable.

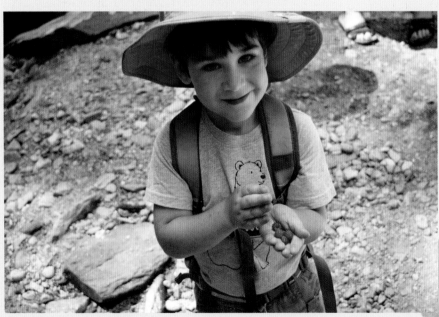

Few things taste better than wild raspberries found along the trail.

PLANTS for TASTING

PLANT	DESCRIPTION
FRUITING TREES	
Mulberry (*Morus rubra*)	Birds and kids love mulberries. (Be careful not to plant the invasive *Morus alba.**)
Pawpaw (*Asimina triloba*)	Grows in moist soil in sun or shade. Produces giant, banana-pear-custard-tasting edible berries in autumn. Loved by possums, raccoons, and people.
Redbud (*Cercis canadensis*)	Edible flowers make a beautiful addition to salads and pancakes.
Serviceberry aka juneberry (*Amelanchier* species)	Delicious blueberry-like berries in June.
Staghorn sumac (*Rhus typhina*)	Berries can be crushed for a tart and delicious lemonade-like drink.
SHRUBS WITH BERRIES (most need more than one plant to produce fruit)	
Blackberry* (*Rubus* species)	Blackberries can cover a fence in a sunny spot. Be sure to ask for a thornless variety. Leaves are edible and medicinal.
Elderberry (*Sambucus canadensis*)	Fast-growing shrub for damp or wet, sunny spots. Berries appear in late summer for making jams, pies, and wine. Elderberries also build immunity and fight colds and sore throats.
Highbush or lowbush blueberry (*Vaccinium* species)	Yummy, filled-with-antioxidant berries—if you can get to them before the birds do! Blueberries also offer striking red fall color.
Huckleberry (*Gaylussacia baccata*)	Grows in dry, acidic soil and does best with a few hours of sun. Like blueberries, huckleberry shrubs turn bright red in the fall. Berries are delicious by the handful or in pancakes, muffins, or pies.
LOW-GROWING BERRIES	
Ground cover raspberry* (*Rubus* 'Formosa Carpet')	This creeper is happy in light shade. It has fuzzy leaves and tiny golden fruit.
Strawberry* (*Fragaria × ananassa*)	Try planting strawberries instead of traditional ground cover for evergreen color all year and delicious fruit in late spring to early summer.

PICKIN' PAW PAW UP PAWS PUT THEM IN YOUR POCKET

*Indicates non-native. All other plants listed are North American natives.

TOUCH THE EARTH EVERY DAY

A wise teacher I know gave this assignment to her homework-hungry kindergartners: Touch the earth every day. It required them to develop a habit—to learn to pause, to be aware, and to notice nature. Touching the earth can be broadly defined in many ways. Sand, soil, water, and mud are essential elements of the earth that should be encountered as often as possible. They offer open-ended play, infinite opportunities for experimentation and creativity, and a softness that is soothing and healing. A tray of sand is a common tool for children's therapists because it is so calming. Raking gravel or sand in a Zen garden is a time-honored meditative pastime. All of these materials are malleable and responsive; they allow us to explore everything from physics and engineering to creativity and art. Playing with these rich sensory materials is deeply engaging, so it is important not only to include them, but to allow children plenty of time to engage with them.

Sand

Depending on how wet or dry it is, sand can be sifted, shaped, smoothed, raked, sculpted, and climbed. It is a raw material for pretending: one minute a birthday cake, the next a tunnel or moat. Raking patterns into soft sand with our fingers requires a light touch. Lifting a heavy bucket of sand exercises the proprioceptive sense, which helps us assess the force required by our body to move an object. A big digging project may require the help of friends, which adds a social dimension and a chance to develop negotiation skills. Textures below the sand are a surprise to uncover. Bury treasures like marbles and gems—colored aquarium gravel paired with a sand sifter works great. A big pile of sand dumped in your play space is a smart investment that offers more diverse play value than any other single element I can think of.

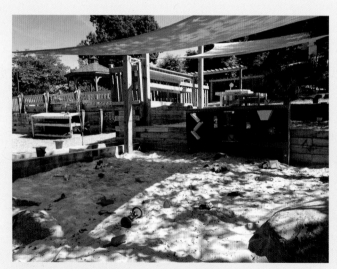

A sandpit is bordered by a tempting sand play wall.

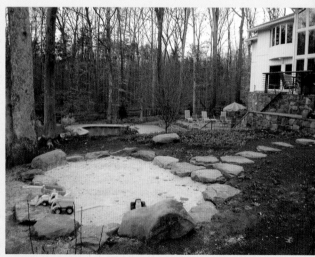

A simple backyard sandpit bordered by boulders and populated with a few toys provides hours of enjoyment.

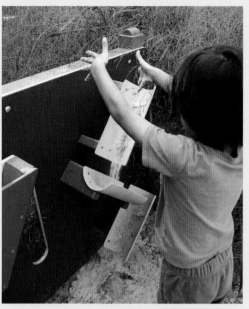

Vertical surfaces outfitted with chutes, wheels, and openings of various sizes help children develop their arms and core muscles as they lift and pour.

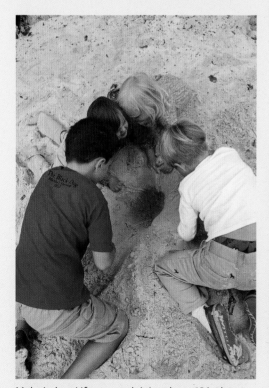

Make it deep! If your sandpit is at least 18 inches, preferably 24, children can do the serious digging they crave.

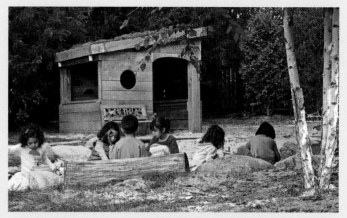

A comfortable sand play area will invite children to linger. It's a place for conversation, relaxing, and hanging out.

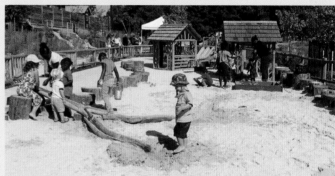

Adding water play elements, as here at Constitution Gardens Park outside Washington, DC, increases the appeal of a sandpit in a child's eyes.

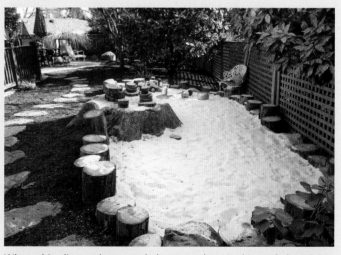

When a big, diseased tree needed to come down in this yard, the owners retained the stump as a work surface and repurposed wood rounds to enclose a backyard sandpit.

CARING FOR SAND

Many people worry about animals around sand, especially cats using the sandpit as a litter box. There does not seem to be any research that supports this fear, so unless you have evidence of a problem, don't be unnecessarily concerned. If there are cats or foxes or other animals using nearby mulch, the dirt under a shrub in your yard, or other parts of your play space, then perhaps they will be drawn to your sand. Motion-triggered water sprayers are one approach to scaring away animal trespassers. Another is to cover the sandpit. Keep in mind that the most important strategy for keeping sand clean is to be sure it has good drainage below, so water doesn't sit in the sand. To that end, always use open mesh, a wire grid, or lattice to cover the sand, not a plastic tarp, because solid plastic closes in moisture. Sand that stays damp for days is a good medium for growing bacteria. Sunshine, fresh air, and good drainage are the best aids in keeping sand clean. Raking out debris such as sticks and rotting leaves on a regular basis helps, too. If your sand is in a public setting, such as a neighborhood park, you will want to check for glass and trash every day before children use the space.

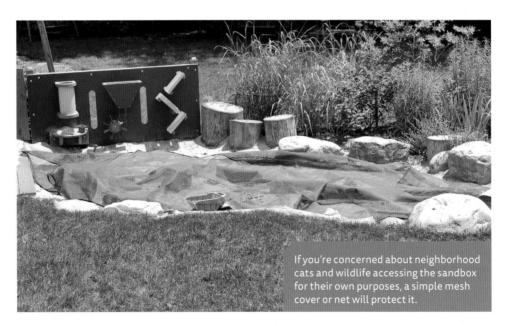

If you're concerned about neighborhood cats and wildlife accessing the sandbox for their own purposes, a simple mesh cover or net will protect it.

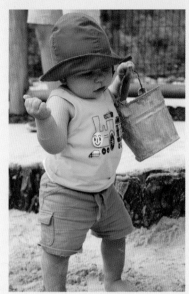

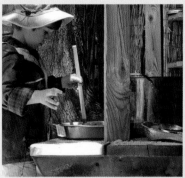

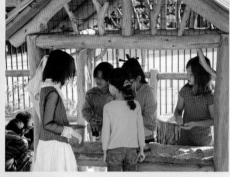

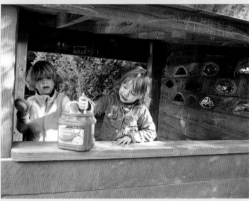

Work surfaces added to a sand play area—pass-through windows, shelves, pretend ovens, stumps, and tables—enhance and sustain play, encourage a variety of body postures, and support social interactions and imagination.

Even toddlers can learn about their bodies and their capabilities by balancing, bending, squatting, lifting, and carrying in sand.

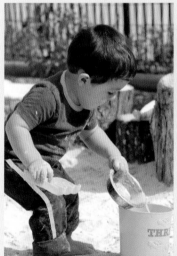

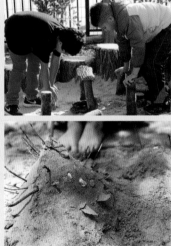

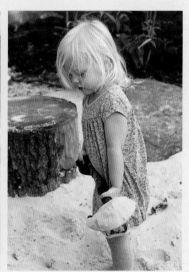

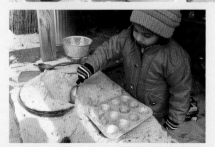

Loose parts in the sand can include containers, kitchenware, digging tools, and tree parts. These enrich sand play and develop imagination, problem solving, and small and large muscles.

A SANDPIT

WHAT YOU'LL NEED

* garden hose or rope
* landscape-marking spray paint
* shovel and digging tools
* coarse gravel to cover the bottom of your sandpit to a depth of 6 to 12 inches
* stumps and logs 12 to 24 inches in diameter (cedar, black locust, maple, and oak work well)
* router or chainsaw
* geotextile fabric the size of the sandpit
* washed play sand or beach sand to fill the sand pit, 18 to 24 inches deep
* wheelbarrow
* small boulders (enough when combined with the stumps and logs to encircle your sandpit)

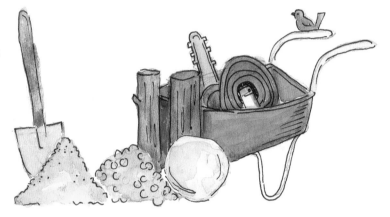

1 Decide on a location for your sand play area. Remember that a shady spot under a tree, while inviting, will be filled with tree roots when you dig out the area, and will result in extra leaves and debris in the sand. If you do choose a space under a tree, try to dig around roots as much as possible. Too much disruption in the critical root zone can kill a tree, sometimes a year or two after the fact. A spot out in the sunshine may be warm on a summer day, but the sunshine will keep the sand dry and prevent the growth of mold that can happen in damp sand.

2 Using garden hose or rope, lay out a pleasing organic shape for your digging area. Think about how many children and adults will be in the area and make it as large as possible. Remember to allow space for the log edging and provide enough sand area for tools, any work surfaces, and busy little bodies.

3 Mark the edge outlines by spray painting them on the ground. Mark both the edge where the sand will end and the outer ring where the log edging will sit. The width of the ring should match the width of your logs, so make the ring about 12 to 24 inches.

4 Dig out the inner area, 24 to 30 inches deep.

5 Dig out the outer ring, 12 inches deep.

6 Fill the bottom 6 to 12 inches of the inner sand area with coarse gravel.

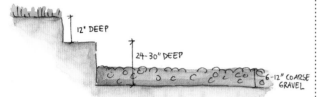

7 Cut stumps 18 to 30 inches tall. Variety is good.

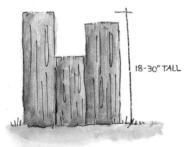

8 Round the top edge of the stumps with a router or bevel with a chainsaw.

9 You can remove the bark or let it fall off naturally, which will happen within weeks or months, depending on the type of wood you use.

10 Set stumps in place along the ring you've prepared. Place them as close together as possible. This may require shaving a little off the sides to get a better fit. They don't need to fit perfectly, but the snugger they are, the less sand will leak out between stumps.

Intersperse some boulders or a horizontal log for variety—this makes the edge of the sandpit a good place for balancing, sitting, or working.

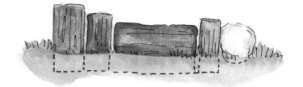

11 Place a layer of geotextile fabric over the gravel and let it wrap up the inside edge of the stumps a few inches. If desired, you can staple it onto the logs, below the height of the eventual top of the sand.

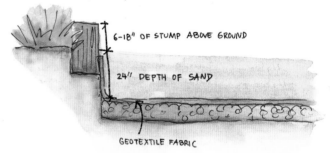

12 Fill the sandpit with sand. Use a wheelbarrow to move sand in, or if your site allows access, have a dump truck back up and dump the sand right into the prepared area. Kids can be in charge of climbing the sand mountain and it will eventually level out. Try to keep the level of the sand about even with the level of the ground outside.

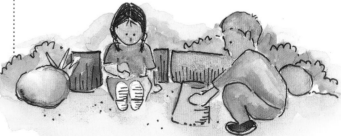

PICKABLE PLANTS

PLANT	DESCRIPTION
GRASSES	
River oats (*Chasmanthium latifolium*)	The oats are dangling jewels which are great fun to pick. Dense roots make river oats also good for holding banks and preventing erosion. (However, they can be difficult to get rid of, so plant carefully.)
ANNUALS	
Zinnia*, cosmos*, marigold*, and pansy*	Each of these easy-to-grow favorites produces two flowers for every one you pick.
PERENNIALS	
Purple coneflower (*Echinacea purpurea*), **black-eyed Susan** (*Rudbeckia hirta*), **tickseed** (*Coreopsis species*), **obedient plant** (*Physostegia virginiana*), **swamp sunflower** (*Helianthus angustifolius*)	All produce abundant flowers for picking.
CONIFERS	
Hemlock (*Tsuga canadensis*), **Douglas fir** (*Pseudotsuga menziesii*), **bald cypress** (*Taxodium distichum*), **dawn redwood*** (*Metasequoia glyptostroboides*), **Eastern red cedar** (*Juniperus virginiana*)	All produce uniquely shaped or berrylike cones that are great for play.
TREES WITH SEED PODS	
Kentucky coffeetree (*Gymnocladus dioicus*), **catalpa** (*Catalpa* family), **redbud** (*Cercis canadensis*), **magnolia** (*Magnolia grandiflora*), **oak** (*Quercus species*)	Kentucky coffeetree, catalpa, and redbud all have long, sometimes rattling seed pods. Magnolia pods don't rattle but are fun to collect. Oak acorns spur the imagination.
SHRUBS WITH BERRIES	
Beautyberry (*Calicarpa americana*)	Beautiful magenta berries aren't delicious to people but aren't toxic and birds love them.
Bayberry (*Myrica pensylvanica*)	Produces waxy berries that were used to make scented candles in colonial days.
Winterberry (*Ilex verticillata*)	A deciduous holly. Plant a male and female to get berries. Avoid eating berries, however; they are mildly toxic.

*Indicates non-native. All other plants listed are North American natives.

Soil

Digging in soil offers a different type of proprioceptive experience than digging in loose sand, because soil can be either light and fluffy or dense and dominated by clay. These textures make soil harder or easier to dig and carry, and give it different colors, textures, and smells. Having real metal shovels and tools along with a place to dig is incredibly satisfying to children. Mixing some sand into the soil of a digging spot can make the soil easier to work and different than digging in either material by itself.

Digging in the earth is an engaging, satisfying activity that exercises the body as well as the mind. There are opportunities for making plans (an underground shelter?), setting goals (how deep can I go?), and imagining stories (is there treasure to be found?). And fascinating studies by bacteriologists tell us that there is another benefit to digging and playing in soil. In addition to building our immune systems and reducing the likelihood of asthma and allergies, there are beneficial bacteria, called *Mycobacterium vaccae*, commonly found in soil, which can help us neurologically. More specifically, when these bacteria come in contact with our skin or are inhaled into our lungs, serotonin is produced in our brain. Serotonin is a neurotransmitter that makes us happy, reduces stress, and improves our ability to learn. No wonder playing in dirt or gardening makes us feel good!

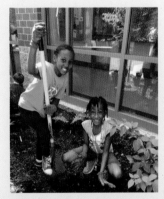

Digging in the dirt exposes us to bacteria that produce serotonin in our brains. Playing in the dirt makes kids (and adults) calm and happy and helps us learn better.

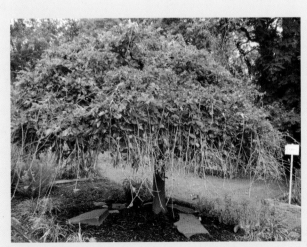

As high as kids could reach, the leaves of this weeping mulberry have been picked clean.

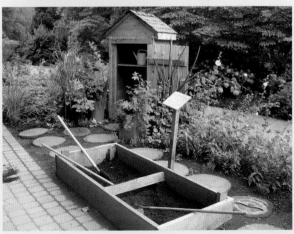

If you're concerned about mess or don't have a dedicated space in your yard, build a digging box filled with soil and real shovels.

Water

Adults often take water for granted, but children never seem to tire of playing with it, especially when it's offered in a play space. Water changes state in mysterious ways for children: liquid freezes solid in cold weather, and in hot summer sun it evaporates and seems to disappear. It can be poured, pumped, sprayed, channeled, and carried in containers. Water always flows downhill, forming puddles and ponds, and sometimes disappears into the ground. Kids who have access to water in their play discover that they can wash with it, drink it, feed plants with it, raise fish in it, swim in it, cook with it, sail on it. There are myriad science lessons that come out of wondering why some things float and others sink. Basins, troughs, and fixed or movable channels can be raised or at ground level, cascading or serpentine. They can be made of hollow logs, concrete with mosaic, clay, or packed earth lined with stone. And they can direct water to flow into sand, where children can create channels, rivers, ponds, moats, and dams. Depending where they live and with the right clothing, children can play with water outdoors throughout the year.

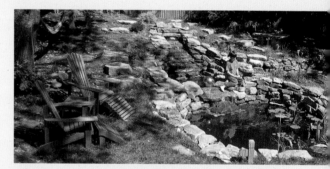

A stream or pond can provide wildlife habitat and endless play value with mud, water, and rocks.

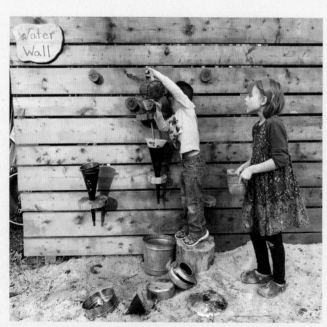

A water wall with rearrangeable funnels, tubes, and even a pulley requires stretching, reaching, lifting, and balancing, plus predicting and planning where the water will go.

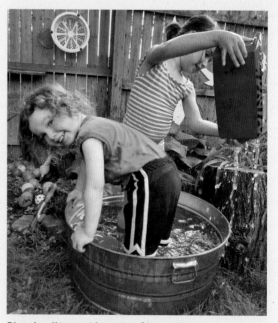

Big tubs allow a wide range of water play experiences. Add a variety of accessories—such as dish soap, plastic toys, colanders, funnels, tubes, and more—to vary the experience.

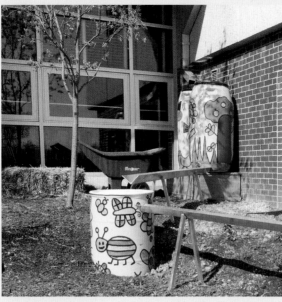

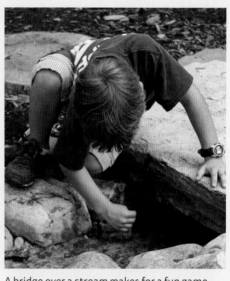

Rainwater is captured in colorful barrels and released to flow down metal troughs and into more barrels. Children can float ping-pong balls in the troughs. Inexpensive plastic gutters can also be used as troughs.

A bridge over a stream makes for a fun game of Pooh Sticks (sticks are dropped into flowing water on the upstream side of the bridge, then players watch to see whose stick emerges first from under the bridge on the downstream side).

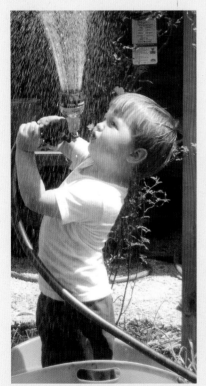

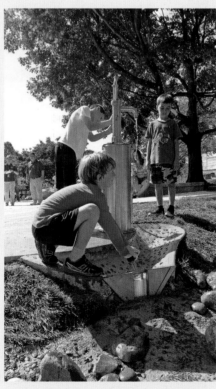

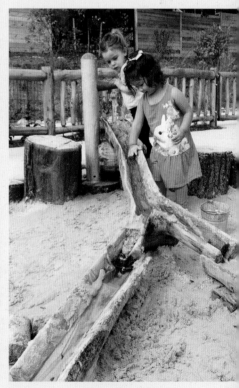

Just by playing with a hose, kids can learn about flow and gravity.

A weir gate allows pumped water to collect in the basin behind it. When the gate is flipped open, water is released with a whoosh.

Water play troughs, such as these versions in locust wood, allow children to experiment with gravity, floating, sinking, and damming up the flow.

PROJECT

A MOSAIC STREAM

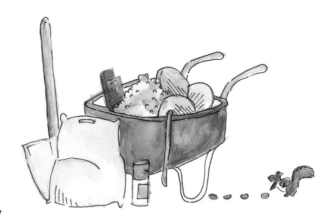

WHAT YOU'LL NEED

* garden hose or rope
* landscape-marking spray paint
* ready-mix concrete (calculate stream's length × width × 3 to 4 inches deep; purchase quantity based on manufacturer's instructions)
* medium gravel (enough to cover bottom of streambed 3 to 4 inches deep)
* hardware cloth
* shovel to mix and scoop concrete
* wheelbarrow or basin for mixing concrete
* water source
* trowel

* level or string line
* assortment of river rocks in different sizes (calculate stream's length × width, guestimate quantity based on rock sizes; staff at source store can help)
* flat-bottomed glass marbles (calculate length × width in inches of stream bottom to be covered in glass marbles; divide that by average size of marble: 1 square inch)

1 Choose a location that slopes slightly downward so water will flow, and be sure the stream ends in an area of your yard that can accommodate water, such as your well-drained sand play area or a rain garden, which is also specifically designed for water to infiltrate easily.

2 Lay out one edge of your stream using a rope or garden hose. Play with it until you get a good curve.

3 Spray paint the curve.

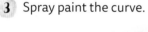

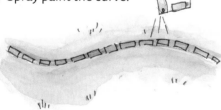

4 To place the opposite bank, measure the width of your stream at intervals across from the first line. Spray a dot of paint about every foot along the opposite edge. (A good width is 18 inches for most of the stream. You may want it to be wider at the mouth where it empties into your sandbox or rain garden.)

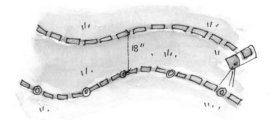

5 Connect all the dots with a smooth line of paint.

6 Dig out the stream to whatever depth you prefer. An average depth of 8 to 12 inches is usually good; 12 to 18 inches in the stream center. Make sure there is a steady slope downward, so water will flow and not puddle up. Use a string line or a level to check this.

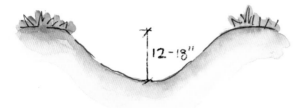

7 Line the streambed with medium gravel about 3 to 4 inches deep at the bottom of the basin. Spread it out so it's even and curves up the sides of the streambed.

8 Lay hardware cloth on top of the gravel. Be sure it's formed into the curves of the streambed.

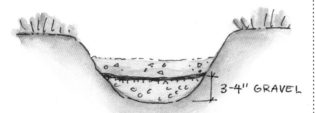

9 For the remaining steps, choose a day when you know you'll have time to complete them all in one day. This part of the project works best with at least two people, one to mix the concrete, and one or more to set the glass beads and stones.

10 Mix up the concrete, one bag at a time.

11 Starting at the top of the stream, pour wet concrete into the streambed, trowel it smooth, and press it up the sides, so it creates the profile you want.

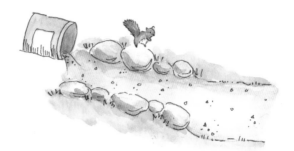

12 Work quickly to set medium and large river rocks along the edge of the stream. Create a line of glass beads down the center that varies in width. You can be playful with this line and imagine what water would do when it flows down the stream. Fill in between the beads and the large rocks with small river rocks. Try not to leave any bare concrete; it won't be very pretty.

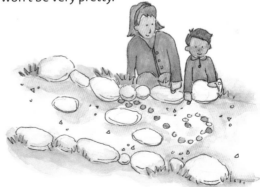

13 Mix the next bag of concrete and pour it into the next section of streambed, troweling away the seam between batches. Continue adding river rocks and glass beads. Repeat as needed to reach the lower end of the streambed.

14 Periodically put a large river rock in the center, or a piece of flat flagstone to create a little step where water will fall.

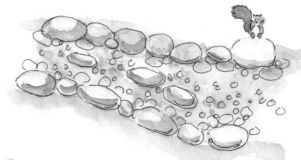

15 Create a wide mouth and a smooth cut edge to the concrete, so water can flow unobstructed into the rain garden or sand area.

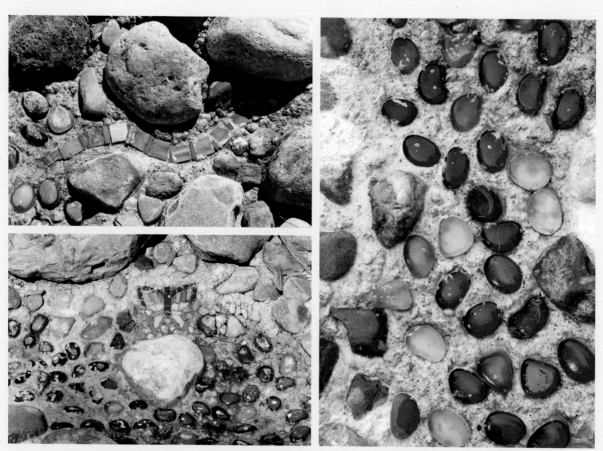

This concrete stream was decorated in collaboration with a mosaic artist and features tiles, glass marbles and beads, and river rocks. The stream is a beautiful addition to the play space, even when water isn't flowing.

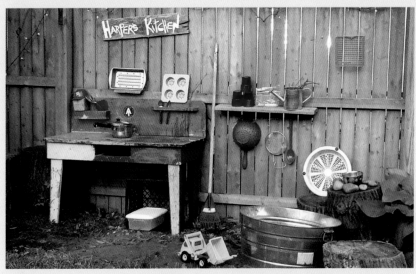

Raid your kitchen or visit a thrift shop to stock a
mud café: pots, pans, measuring cups, cupcake tins,
colanders, ladles, scoops, and other utensils are just
a few possible items.

Mud

When soil and water are combined, the play value
grows exponentially. Now there is the opportunity to create soups and potions, to build structures out of earth, to paint faces and immerse
toes or bodies in a mooshy-squooshy, spa-like
mud bath. Children have differing degrees of
comfort with the sensory intensity of mud. Be
respectful of this, and never push a child beyond
their comfort zone, but do expose them to mud
and messiness from an early age. The more mud
and unusual textures become familiar to children, the more likely kids are to feel comfortable
touching and interacting, and reaping the benefits of those important sensory experiences.

A mud pit can, for the bravest of parents, be a
designated portion of a play space. Loosen some
dirt in one corner of your yard and run the hose
there. Kids can play in bathing suits or under-
wear, or, in colder weather, wear waterproof gear
over clothing. Having a hose, towels, and dry
clothes at the ready for cleanup is helpful.

A mud café is the perfect place for pretending
and experimenting with "recipes" and

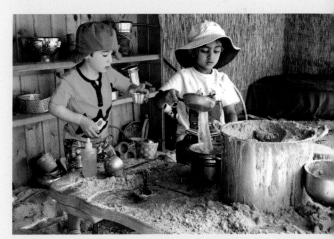

Mud cafés encourage all sorts of experiments and
activities that get children in the habit of being curious
about processes.

concoctions. Because it involves work surfaces
and containers instead of total immersion as
with a mud pit, it is somewhat more manageable
and can be used almost year-round. The ideal
mud café involves a work surface and some low

walls or shelving to make the space feel enclosed. The pass-through windows on many of the playhouses shown in this book are ideal for mud kitchens. There can be a vertical panel (like a fence) for hooks to hang containers and kitchen utensils, along with some storage shelves. A basin for mixing water and later for cleaning up is a good idea.

This is a place for experiencing textures, using imagination, and even for some early literacy. Adding a clipboard and paper or a chalkboard allows kids to document their "recipes." To make mud, you can use soil from your yard or bagged topsoil from a garden center. Wet sand is similar to mud and offers great play value.

The joys of mud are becoming more widely acknowledged. There is now even International Mud Day (created by the World Forum for Early Childhood Care and Education), held on or around June 29 each year. You and your family or community can register your events and share photos of your International Mud Day antics on social media. The pumper truck from the Ithaca, New York, fire department visits the Anarchy Zone adventure playground at the Ithaca Children's Garden and sprays freshly dug soil with water to kick off that town's celebration of International Mud Day.

FEASTING IN NATURE

My mother could be reliably counted on to comment that "food always tastes better outside" whenever we grilled burgers on our little hibachi or had sandwiches on the beach. We teased her about it, but she was right. Whether it is a juicy tomato picked and eaten warm off the vine, a charred-outside-but-fluffy-inside potato roasted over a campfire after a day of hiking, or crunchy apples, crusty bread, and sharp cheese at an outdoor concert, eating outside seems to strip away distractions and connect us to the flavors, the juiciness, and the aromas of our food, and to nature, in a visceral way.

I recommend that children eat outside as often as possible. To really immerse yourself in the drippiness of a hunk of watermelon, you have

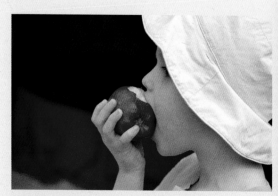

Eating an apple straight from the tree delivers a special kind of satisfaction.

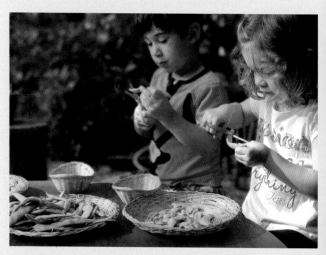

Young chefs practice scissor skills while shelling beans for lunch.

to be outdoors. Having a stash of snacks in your pocket, ready to go to whenever hunger hits, makes a person feel in charge, competent, and ready for anything.

A place to eat outside can be a bench, a blanket laid on the ground, or a table and chairs. A water source makes washing veggies or sticky hands much easier, whether it's a simple bucket of warm water, a sink hooked up to plumbing, or something in between. Creating outdoor storage space for grilling tools, a harvest basket, a knife for slicing watermelon, and other necessities makes spur-of-the-moment outdoor meals more likely.

Fire

The discovery of fire is said to be one of the things that makes humans unique among the creatures who share our planet. Adding heat to our food transforms it in taste, texture, color, smell and sometimes in digestibility. By adding a source of heat to our outdoor space, we widen the variety of what we can eat, and add a deeper layer of sustenance to our time outside.

A solar oven is a remarkable device that can harness and concentrate the heat of the sun in ways that are sometimes surprising. A basic cardboard box, covered in aluminum foil with some insulation and a sheet of glass can actually boil water, cook a pan of brownies, or roast a pot of stew.

Making an outdoor oven out of cob (soil, sand, water, and straw) can be an undertaking for the whole family—or the neighborhood. The book *Build Your Own Earth Oven* (2007) is a great resource for instructions. A cob oven becomes a place for gathering or for feeding a group. A fire is started inside the oven, which heats up

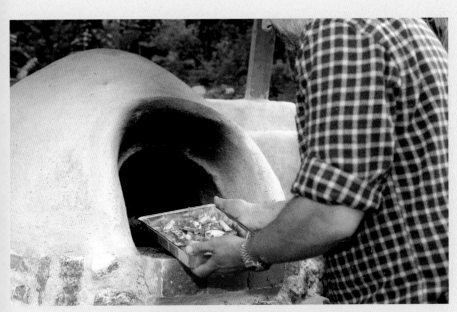

Homegrown vegetables are ready for roasting in this hand-built cob oven.

the masonry. That stored heat slowly releases and can cook pizzas, loaves of bread, vegetables, or meats.

A simple fire circle can become a gathering place that invites us to stay outside after the sun sets, by providing light and warmth and safety. Sitting by an evening bonfire in any season invites storytelling, music, and relaxed conversation. Watching the stars come out and the sparks of the fire rise up slows down the pace of life and brings us closer to our ancient, primitive selves. Cooking around a campfire is a joyful experience. Every child can have their own stick for roasting a hotdog or a marshmallow. What could be better?

Vegetable gardening as nature play

When children help plant, care for, and harvest food, they are much more likely to taste new things. Many a parent has been surprised by the enthusiasm of picky young eaters to pluck and sample fresh peas from the vine, especially if the legumes have been grown by the kids themselves.

A vegetable garden can be in the ground or in containers on your balcony. If you live someplace without room for planting, find out about local community gardens. In addition to providing a green oasis in the city and a place for children to grow their own vegetables and flowers, community gardens can be a place to gather with like-minded people and learn from each other. Weeding and using garden tools build important muscles in children's arms and hands, which help develop fine motor skills such as writing, drawing, and cutting. If you build a cold frame, you can even extend the harvest season.

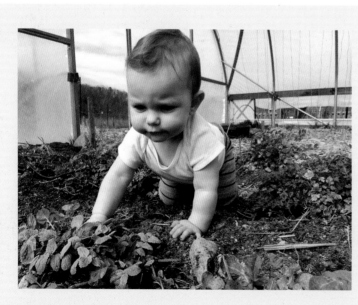

Connecting with plants and soil can begin early. Babies soak up sensory experiences in the garden.

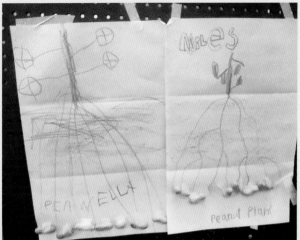

Talk with your children about all the parts of a plant as together you plant, nurture, harvest, and eat from your own garden.

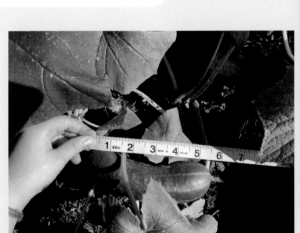

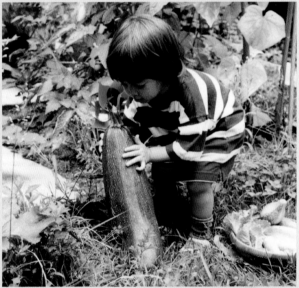

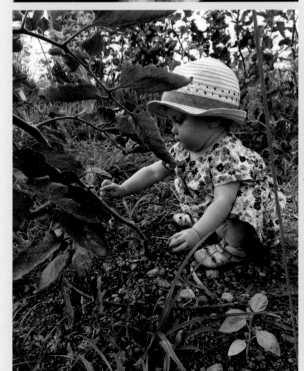

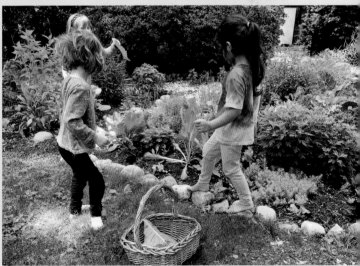

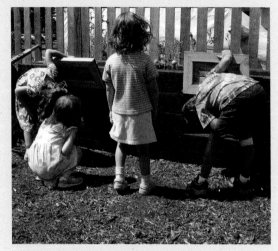

Plexiglass viewing windows allow a peek at root vegetables (potatoes, radishes, carrots, even peanuts) growing underground.

It's also fun to think about how different parts of plants provide food for people, depending on the season. In the spring there are tender new leaves such as lettuce and spinach and stems such as asparagus and bamboo shoots. As summer settles in, we have flowers—broccoli, cauliflower and artichokes; fruits such as zucchini, tomatoes, cucumbers, and peppers; plus seeds such as beans and peas. During winter, we are able to enjoy the leaves of hardy greens such as collards, kale, cabbage, and chard, as well as root vegetables that were harvested earlier, but which store well and continue to offer nutritional benefits. Keep a list, maybe on the kitchen chalkboard, about seasonal vegetables you'd like to try growing.

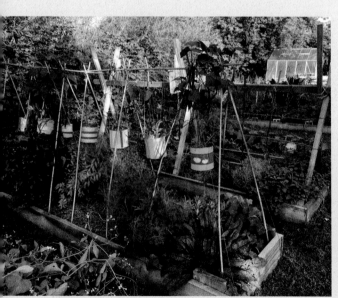
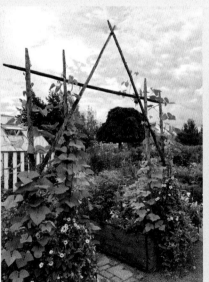
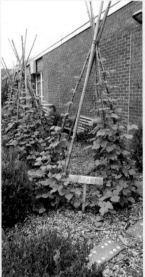

Raised beds can be enhanced with vertical structures to support vines. Divide beds with string to mark separate sections for each child.

RAINBOW GARDENING

You can grow an assortment of colorful edibles any which way, with a harvest that can make a rainbow on your plate. Or, if you have enough space, beds can be arranged in concentric, arching rows, each row planted with foods of the same color, to create a rainbow. The pot of gold at the end of the rainbow can be a bed of yellow pollinator-attracting plants: spring daffodils, summer sneezeweed (*Helenium*) and sunflower (*Helianthus*), and autumn goldenrod (*Solidago*). In any case, plant some of each color so you can eat that rainbow!

EAT-THE-RAINBOW FRUITS and VEGETABLES

COLOR	EDIBLE PLANT
RED	Tomatoes, red peppers, radishes, beets, raspberries, strawberries, watermelon
ORANGE	Orange peppers, pumpkins, butternut squash, carrots, cantaloupe, peaches
YELLOW	Summer squash, banana peppers, wax beans, corn, yellow tomatoes, pears, yellow raspberries
GREEN	Lettuce, zucchini, green beans, kale, broccoli, brussels sprouts, cucumbers, peas, apples, kiwi berries, pawpaws
BLUE AND PURPLE	Blue potatoes, chard, eggplant, purple cabbage, hyacinth bean, blueberries, grapes, plums, blackberries, mulberries, serviceberries, purple onions
WHITE	Cauliflower, garlic, onions, potatoes, turnips

AN HERB SPIRAL

Eagle Scouts created this herb spiral, a project that takes about half a day. It's a perfect project for recycled stone or old bricks.

WHAT YOU'LL NEED

* string
* approximately ⅓ pallet of stone for a 3-foot-diameter spiral
* newspaper for bottom of spiral
* sandy mix of topsoil or potting soil to fill the bed
* assortment of herbs for planting
* shovel

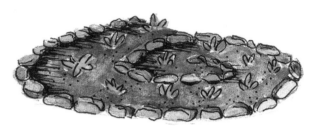

1 Mark a circle on the ground with string, approximately 3 feet in diameter, to locate the herb spiral.

2 Set one course of wall stones around the perimeter of the circle. Clear the area inside the circle of as much grass and plant material as possible.

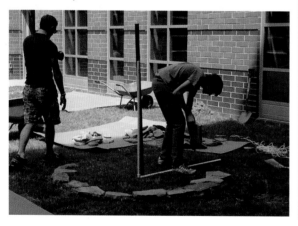

3 Cover the area inside the circle with newspaper.

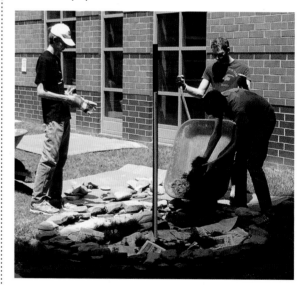

4 Add an additional course of stone around the perimeter and create the stone spiral inside the circle.

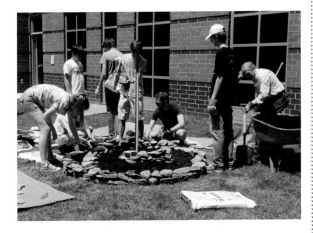

5 Create a soil mound spiraling inward.

6 The herb spiral has microclimates: driest on top, wettest at the bottom, partly shaded on the north, full sun on the south side. Plant deep-rooted, dry-soil, and sun-loving herbs, such as rosemary and lavender, on top. Thyme, sage, oregano, and tarragon can be placed on the sides. Herbs that like cooler, wetter soil, such as parsley, chives, and basil, will be happiest around the bottom.

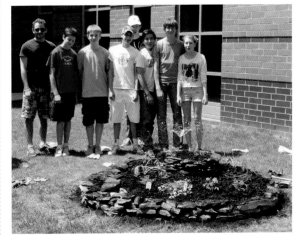

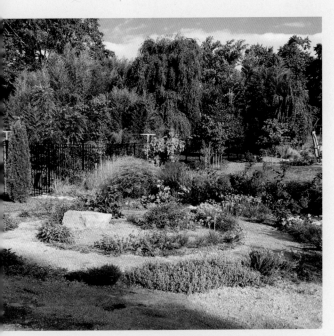

Consider enlisting your kids to help build an herb spiral dedicated to the flavors of your family's heritage. This spiral herb garden at Constitution Gardens is planted with herbs from around the world. The goal is to connect immigrant visitors to the tastes and scents of home.

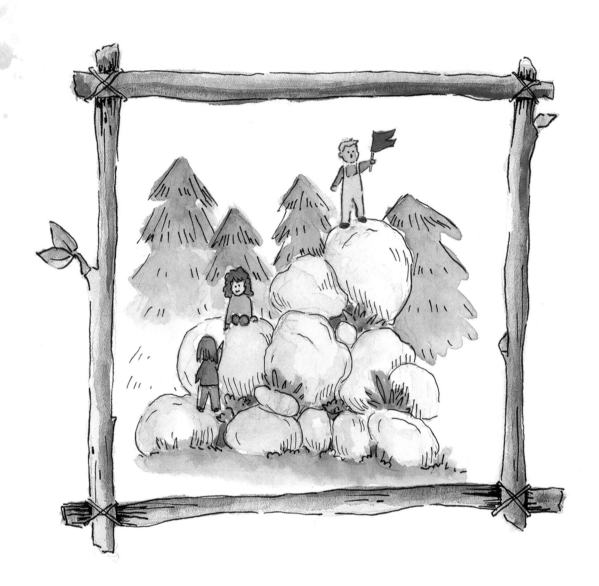

CHALLENGING BODIES

"As safe as necessary, not as safe as possible."
—from the *Risk in Play and Learning Declaration*,
developed by the International School Grounds Alliance

When children use their bodies actively, they learn *to* move and learn *by* moving. We can sculpt the earth into hills and valleys, add tree parts and boulders, and create an up-and-down-scape that invites adventurous play. In this space, children develop balance, endurance, strength, coordination, and confidence. A diverse environment with variety in topography, vegetation, and materials helps children learn to control their bodies in the world and to control the objects in their world. For healthy physical and brain development, children should be spending a significant portion of each day engaged in active, unstructured free play. As described by Angela Hanscom in *Balanced and Barefoot* (2016), school-age children need three to four hours a day of active play, and younger children, who are primarily sensory-motor learners, need even more—up to eight hours a day using their bodies.

In the 1910s, Olympic athlete Jim Thorpe reportedly tried to spend a day imitating every movement of a toddler and collapsed from exhaustion before the day was done. He could not keep up with the range of movement and energy exerted by his baby counterpart. Young children have hundreds of muscles they must strengthen and learn to control, and they are driven to do just that. To try and curtail that motion is to stifle a fundamental need.

IRREGULAR, NATURAL MATERIALS

Natural materials can be arranged to support all sorts of adventurous activities: slopes, boulders, and trees for climbing; trails and open spaces for running; logs and wobbly rocks for balancing; hills for rolling and sliding down; vines, bars, ropes, and branches for hanging and swinging from. There are also many objects found in nature—big and small, heavy and light—to

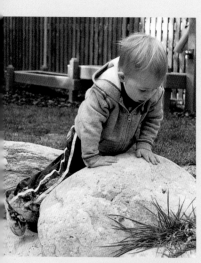

When children move their bodies around an irregularly shaped object, they learn what they are capable of and improve their motor skills.

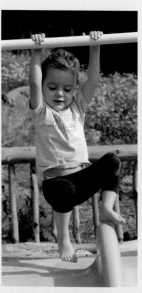

Hanging allows a child to feel her body swing in space.

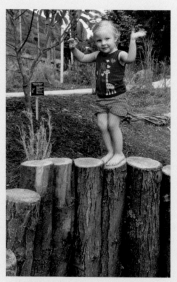

Balancing develops muscle coordination, strength, and (not surprisingly) balance.

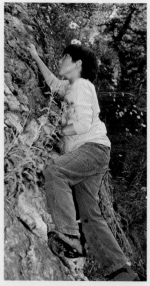

Scaling a vertical rock face takes focus and coordination.

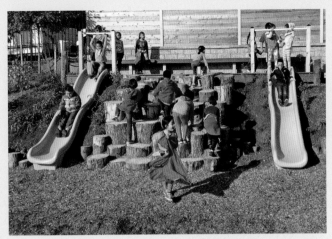

This hill has been enhanced with embankment slides and a stump scramble to make it an inviting space for active play.

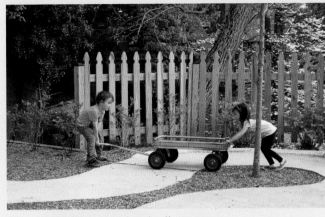

Kids work together to push and pull a wagon.

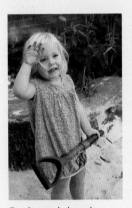

Real metal shovels allow serious digging.

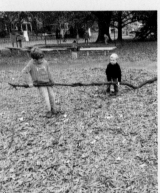

Cooperation makes it possible to move a heavy branch.

push, pull, grasp, lift, carry, drag, throw, and kick. Abundant time and access to active free play and opportunities to crawl, climb, throw, lift, push, pull, and dig allow children to develop core muscles (back, chest, stomach, and neck) and other muscles of the upper body.

These activities help kids learn what they are capable of, and that helps them know themselves better. They discover where they will fit, what they can reach by stretching, how they can bend, what will hold them, and how to balance. Unlike on manufactured, uniformly sized and shaped play equipment, active play in nature requires children to pay attention and adapt their hands and feet to irregularly shaped and spaced branches and uneven boulders.

When children discover something they can't do, it can be an opportunity to practice and achieve a goal. Balancing and walking across a log over a stream, pulling oneself up onto a big boulder, or climbing to the next highest branch of a tree are milestones that build confidence. Progressive levels of difficulty built into a play element are known as graded challenges and make the space appealing to children at different ages over time. Natural play spaces are full of them and it is part of what keeps nature more interesting over time than static, built pieces.

These activities and the skills they promote help kids move safely through the world and reduce their risk of injuries throughout life. Real (metal not plastic) shovels and dirt for digging, heavy things like logs and rocks of different sizes and shapes, buckets to fill and carry with water, sand, and stone all require kids to work hard. Hard work builds muscles and bones, a strong core, and stable joints.

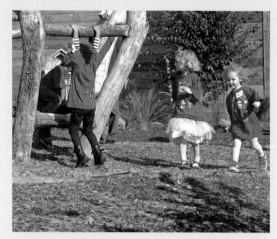

When the environment is rich and varied, kids stay busy and physically active.

In a natural play space, the way the components support different areas of child development are all connected and intertwined. For example, working together with friends to move a heavy log which is being used as a bench in the mud café requires social skills to negotiate, imagination to come up with the scenario, as well as muscles, coordination, and a good proprioceptive sense to be able to actually execute the task. A rugged, challenging terrain asks children to walk, run, leap, balance, crawl, stretch, and climb, and one activity naturally segues into the next. The variety of natural terrain is what keeps children engaged, involved, and motivated.

Research from the University of Tennessee, Knoxville, confirms that children who play in play spaces that incorporate natural elements like boulders, logs, and plants tend to be more active than those who play on traditional playgrounds with metal and brightly colored equipment. This surprising fact may be because of the variety and constant change that go with natural play spaces. Active play in a natural play space is often combined with imaginative play.

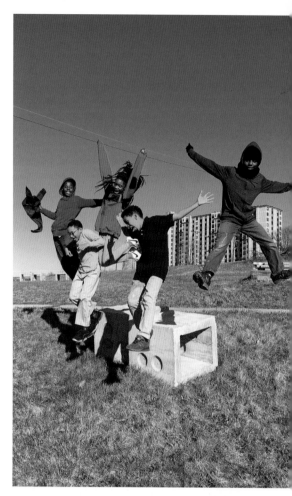

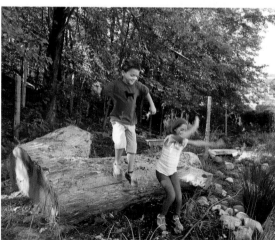

THE SiMPLE ACT OF JUMPiNG

To appreciate the complexity of what is happening as children play, consider this explanation of the seemingly simple act of jumping, by Anita Rui Olds, in "From cartwheels to caterpillars: The child's need for motion outdoors," that appeared in the *Human Ecology Forum* in 1980:

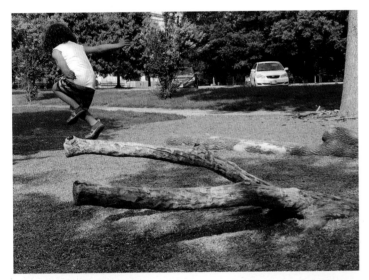

A fundamental aspect of jumping is the material jumped in or upon and the knowledge about the properties of materials and objects that comes from moving and interacting with the physical environment. Will the surface withstand your impact? Will it throw you back, absorb you, tear, rebound, or stretch? It matters whether you jump into something hard or soft, into water, sand, hay, or snow. You can also jump onto something such as a board, or over something such as a rope or a crack in the sidewalk. You can jump to different heights, and across or over things that may be still or in motion. You can jump on flat surfaces or ones that are inclined. You can jump through things like hoops. You can even jump in a seated position by sitting on a ball or an inner tube and bouncing. All these are variations of one simple experience, jumping.

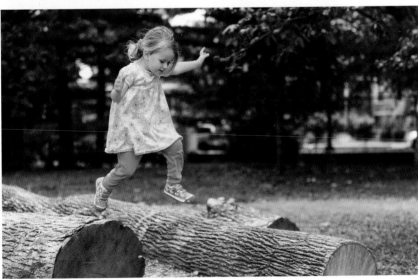

Jumping off requires children to anticipate the distance and how it will feel to land in order to prepare their bodies to stay upright. Sand, wood chips, earth, grass, or another log all feel different. Each requires a specific response.

Elements for babies and toddlers

Small children must move to learn and grow. But before they are mobile, infants need safe places to lie (especially when older siblings are around) and interesting things to gaze at, focus on, and follow with their eyes. The outdoors is a perfect place for this, as birds cavort, busy siblings play, and even light breezes provide intriguing movement to watch.

As the process of developing coordination and body awareness progresses, it's less stressful for parents if a child's environment is designed to allow free and safe movement. Babies who are learning to move will thrive with a variety of surfaces; only moderate changes in level are needed for rolling, creeping, crawling, and toddling. Balance safety with a child's need to explore by anchoring anything that could tip. Add barriers only where safety dictates.

For crawlers and toddlers, many of the natural elements described for older kids will work if they are simpler in form and smaller in scale. Places to go in, out, over, and around provide invitations for crawlers and toddlers to navigate. For infants at the pulling-to-stand stage, bars mounted at about 15 to 18 inches high are a good support for cruising. Toddlers like variety, so there should be open places for roaming and cozy, enclosed places to nestle.

The sensory experiences young children are able to soak up outdoors in the first months of life contribute important building blocks to their development. Providing outside time and an abundance of natural elements goes a long way,

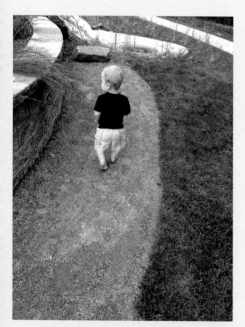

Gravel underfoot, grass to examine, a wall for navigation: sensory input from many channels.

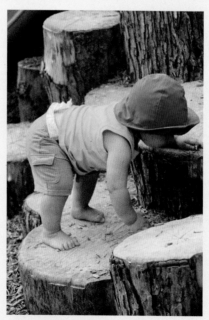

Small conquests offer big rewards for developing bodies.

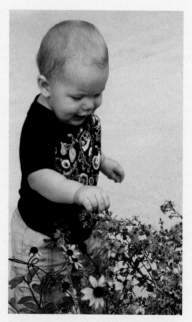

Babies are sensory-motor learners. Touching things that have caught their attention is satisfying.

even at the earliest ages, toward long-term mental, physical, and emotional health.

SURFACES

The surface that children stand upon is the first ingredient in creating a physically challenging and richly engaging play space. What's underfoot can (and should) include a variety of materials, such as boardwalks, mown grass, mulch pathways, hard stone, and stepping stones that create intricate paths for following. There can be elements that encourage the use of alternating feet, unevenness that calls for children to be aware, and soft surfaces like gravel or sand that give way and exercise foot and leg muscles. There can be steps, ramps, and arched bridges that call for navigating grade changes and that exercise one set of muscles going up and another on the descent. Surfaces that are varied and surprising, that require effort to navigate and balance, add a complexity which stimulates hungry brains.

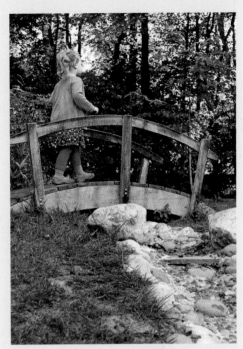

An arched bridge means navigating a curved surface.

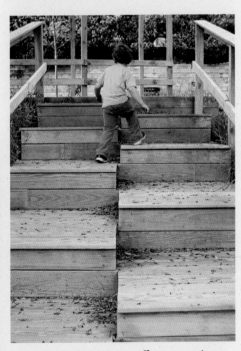

This alternate leg staircase offers two options: walk up on one side or the other taking very big steps, or walk up the center and use both sets of steps together. The center route has smaller gaps, but it requires using alternate legs—a developmental milestone that usually happens sometime during the preschool years.

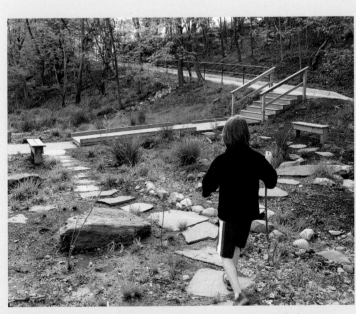

Uneven surfaces require kids to pay attention and maintain balance.

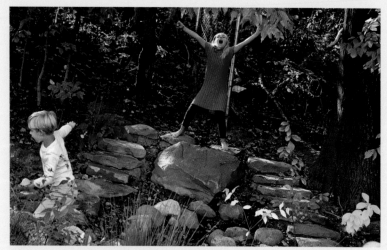

Uneven boulder steps lead up, around, and down this hillside, helping kids develop their sense of balance.

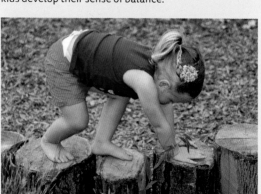

Bare hands and feet work together to scramble and balance.

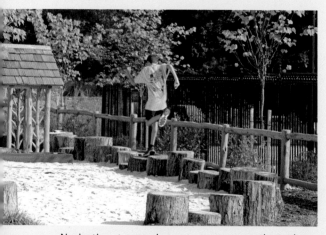

Navigating at a speedy pace over uneven paths, rocks, or stumps requires quick decisions and the ability to accommodate changing terrain.

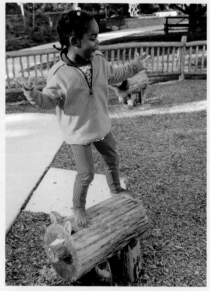

Children need to go barefoot as much as possible, to develop the muscles of their feet, ankles, and legs. You can create a barefoot-specific area and include loose, solid, soft, hard, smooth, bumpy, wobbly, firm, flat, and rounded surfaces.

Safety considerations

It is important to balance safety with the opportunity for children to learn the actual properties of objects, which means knowing that in most places, the ground is hard. Use soft, natural surfaces under spaces intended for climbing to minimize serious injuries. Rubber surfacing may seem like a good choice, but is actually worrisome for a few reasons: the way it holds heat risks not only burning the skin, but also raising the surrounding air temperature, which can actually add to the urban heat island effect. As a petroleum product, rubber also carries the risk of toxicity, and its bounciness can confuse children's developing understanding of the way real ground feels. Around a tree or fallen tree intended for climbing, add wood chips (with good drainage below if it is a place that could get waterlogged).

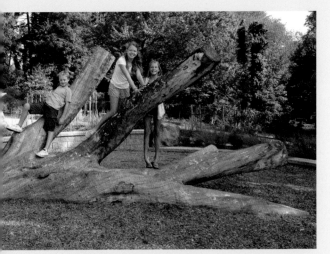
This fallen tree is surrounded by a soft bed of high-quality hardwood chips.

Engineered wood fiber is a type of wood chip that is precisely cut so that chips can be compacted to be relatively wheelchair accessible while still providing a soft landing.

Helpful information and guidelines can be found in the Consumer Product Safety Commission (CPSC) *Outdoor Home Playground Safety Handbook* and the CPSC *Public Playground Safety Handbook*, available at CPSC.gov.

Accommodating riding toys

If your area will include riding toys, think about pathways that meander as far as possible through the space and that contain different textures to make the journey interesting. Short pathways soon become boring. Dead ends, especially without a turnaround, can be frustrating. With riding toys, children can experience rolling, coasting, pushing, pedaling, alternating feet, and steering. Adding varied trails to follow, tunnels to enter and exit, dips and rises in the path, sharp turns, and a few bumps will help riders stay engaged. What I call a "shunnel" (a combined shed and tunnel) is a valuable accessory to the riding area. (More on shunnels later.)

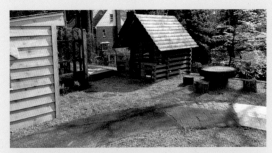
Different textures in the trail create changing sounds and vibrations when pedaled over.

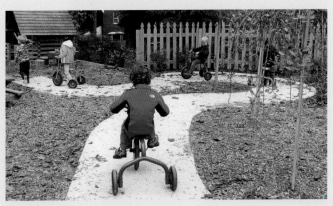
Trikes pass through a shunnel (shed plus tunnel).

A tight loop challenges pedaling and steering.

LANDFORMS

By sculpting the earth we can create interesting undulations in terrain: high and low places, bumps, mounds, berms, ridges, slopes, terraces, steps, holes, ditches, swales, caves, and tunnels. All of these are great ways to add play value to your yard, but hills in particular give children a new view of the world.

Hills

Unlike play equipment, a hill provides elevation without the risk of falling a great distance, so it doesn't require special surfacing. A hill is also a wonderful place to experiment with gravity. Rolling balls, logs, or even wagons and carts down a hill can be very exciting. Pushing, pulling, or carrying those items up the hill is a rewarding challenge. Rolling yourself down a hill helps develop the vestibular sense, which is important in balancing and moving safely. A hill can be as simple as a pile of dirt, sand, mulch, gravel, or meadowy slope, providing a great deal of play value for a very small investment.

When my children were little and we lived in a community that was under construction I learned the importance of mounds. There was always a load of something—fill dirt, topsoil,

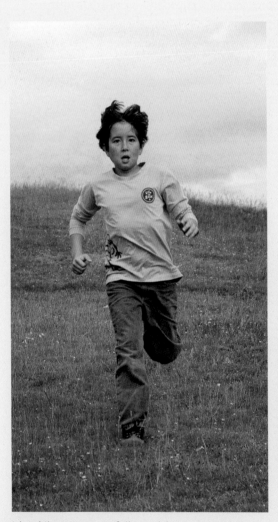

It's exhilarating to run full speed down a grassy hill (with shoes or barefoot).

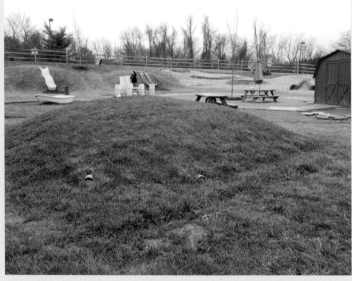

This little hill (with bigger hills in the background) is called the "ant hill." It has a network of interconnected PVC pipes woven throughout. It's easy to drop balls down the pipes—and more challenging to predict where they will come out.

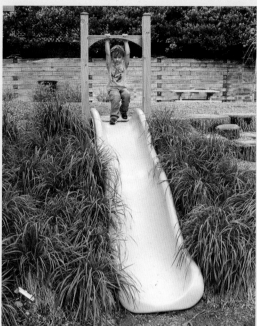
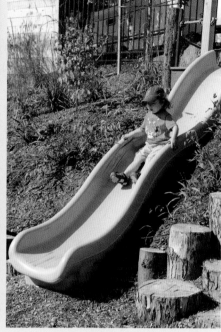

Grasses and other plants add appealing texture and stability to hills with slides.

sand, mulch, or gravel—being delivered. I was fascinated by what a magnet these little mountains of materials were to children of all ages. These piles provided opportunities for digging, tunneling, and engineering. They also gave the neighborhood children a high spot with a view that allowed them to survey their domain, understand the space from a different vantage point, and assess what was happening socially.

Remember that scale is different for a child, too. Places that seemed so big when we were small are revealed through adult eyes to be lower, closer together, and generally less imposing than we recall. It doesn't take much of a hillock to occupy a small child for a long time.

A hill can be a simple dirt pile, but bare dirt hills get worn down by gravity, rain, and lots of little footsteps, sometimes known as kid erosion. Impermanence is fine and adds to the interest

of the space. However, you may decide that you want to maintain the hill and have it become a long-term asset in your space. Embellishing with plants, boulders, steps, ramps, ropes or even a slide will all help to extend the life of a hill. Each of these will add a new dimension by providing challenging alternatives for getting up or down— scrambling using hands and feet on rough boulders, balancing on uneven stump steps, or using upper body muscles with a rope to pull oneself up a steep ramp.

A mowed grassy slope is very inviting as a place to lie or roll or gather with friends. Grass will help to hold the soil in place but is subject to being worn down by little feet. If you absolutely must have grass, know that it survives longer when it is regularly irrigated. Ornamental grasses and other plants with deep root systems are very helpful in preventing erosion on hills.

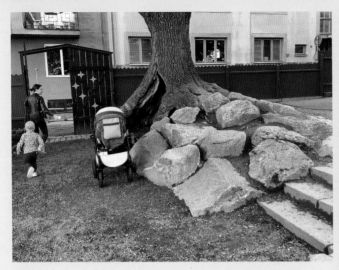

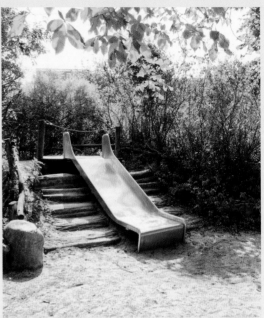

Timber steps and boulders help preserve small hills from erosion.

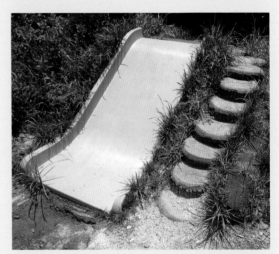

Steps made of tree cookies and a short slide wide enough for two were big hits in this toddler playground.

A slide is a great way to enhance an existing hillside, or it can be added to a hill you build by piling and compacting soil. A slide can be straight or curved, wavy or smooth, big enough for one or wide enough for two. There are lots of different ways to go down the slide, and each one gives a child the opportunity to learn different things about how to control their body as it moves through space. Going up a slide offers a valuable climbing challenge, so don't prohibit that experience unequivocally. Instead, for safety, if there is more than one slide in a play space, designate one for going up, or set aside times when the direction is reversed on the slide. A slide can be made of concrete, wood, metal, or even clay, but in the spaces I design, it is one of the only exceptions to the no-plastic rule. Plastic slides in light colors stay cooler and are never splintery or sharp. You'll need adequate clearance for the slide, a flat space to sit and enter the slide at the top, and a landing zone of six feet of clear space with safety surfacing at the bottom. There should be at least one way to get up the hill, and plants to hold the soil on the hill in place. Slides can be recycled from playground equipment or they can be purchased for the site and installed into the embankment.

PROJECT

A HILLSIDE SLIDE

WHAT YOU'LL NEED

* post hole digger or shovel
* slide of your choice
* 4-by-4-inch posts
* 1 bag ready-mix concrete for each post
* hardware to attach slide to posts
  (purchase hardware to fit slide holes)
* flat rock or large tree cookie at least the width
  of the slide × 2 to 3 feet deep
* safety surfacing (sand, wood chips, or rubber mats)

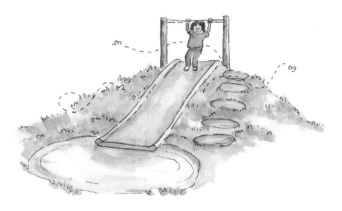

* 2-by-4-inch piece of lumber, or a bar (for crosspiece)
* stumps or boulders for steps
* plants for any bare spots on the hillside

1. In the Northern Hemisphere, slides should always face north unless the hill is well shaded. South-facing slides can get dangerously hot in the afternoon sun.

2. Decide the length of slide you need, depending on the height of the hill.

3. The slide should be set at an angle of between 30 and 35 degrees to work for a range of ages.

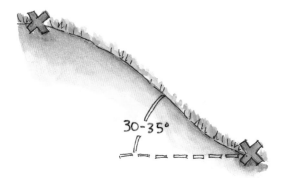

30–35°

4. Set the slide in place on the hill and mark where the top and bottom edges will go.

5. If the angle of the hill needs to be adjusted, it is best to dig out some of the hill, not build up, because whatever soil you try to add will be particularly susceptible to erosion.

6. Follow the installation instructions from the slide manufacturer, if you have them. If you don't have instructions, one way to install the slide securely is to bolt the top and bottom of the slide onto 4-by-4-inch posts that measure at least 30 inches tall.

7. Dig holes in the spots where you want the top and bottom of the slide to be, and set the posts in place.

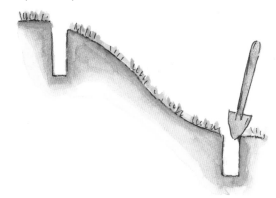

8 Mix and add concrete to the post holes to anchor the posts in the ground. Once the concrete is dry, use hardware to attach the slide to bottom posts.

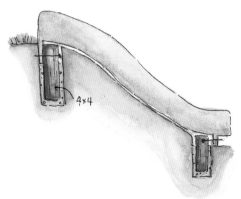

9 A sit-down bar can be constructed by setting a post on either side of the top entry of the slide and adding a bar or wood beam between them at about 30 to 36 inches above the top of the slide. This will prevent kids from riding their bikes or skateboards down the slide.

10 Leave a gap of between 1 and 3 inches between the top of the slide and the posts, so hood strings can't get stuck here as children slide down.

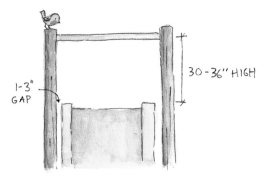

11 You can set a large tree cookie, a large flat rock, or even build a little platform at the top to provide a stable surface for easy entry onto the slide.

12 Make natural steps using stumps, logs, tree cookies, or flat boulders. Children will most likely want to go up following the most direct path, so to avoid an eroded dirt path alongside the slide, locate the steps as close to the slide as possible. Be sure they are low enough that they don't extend above the lip of the slide anywhere along the route to the top of the hill. If space allows, have more than one way up, using different materials, spaced out over the hillside.

13 Plant in between the paths to help avoid erosion. Edging can help protect the plants and soil from foot traffic.

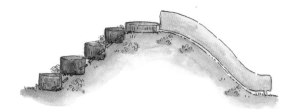

14 At the bottom, create a landing zone of safety surfacing (sand, wood chips, or rubber mats) at least 6 inches deep, and keep the area clear. Rubber mats are not ideal, as mentioned earlier, but their advantage is that they will not shift with foot traffic. Loose fill will need to be raked back into place regularly to avoid a big, water-collecting pit at the bottom of the slide. (Although sliding into water can be its own fun, when it's intentional.)

Plants to Help Prevent Hillside Erosion

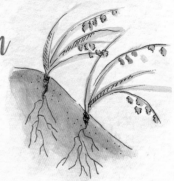

The grasses of the American prairie are known for their deep and extensive roots, which held the soil and helped build the rich farmlands of the central United States. Grasses native to riverbanks are also known for strong roots that hang on through drought and deluge. Any of the grasses listed here, once established, will form thick root systems to help avoid or stop erosion on your hill.

Bottlebrush grass (*Elymus hystrix*) Good for shady slopes.

Indian grass (*Sorghastrum nutans*) Low-growing prairie grass with late summer blooms 3 to 5 feet tall.

Mexican feather grass (*Nassella tenuissima*) Very soft and strong. Good in full sun.

Prairie dropseed (*Sporobolus heterolepis*) Soft grass grows 2 to 3 feet tall in full sun.

River oats (*Chasmanthium latifolium*) Good for sun or shade; 2 to 3 feet tall.

Switchgrass (*Panicum virgatum*) Tough, easy-care grass that grows 3 to 6 feet tall in full sun.

Tussock sedge (*Carex stricta*) Great for a wet, sunny hill.

The following plants are known to spread and colonize, and thus work well when planted on hills.

Green and gold (*Chrysogonum virginianum*) Low-growing ground cover with yellow flowers in spring. Does well in shade.

'Gro-Low' sumac (*Rhus aromatica* 'Gro-Low') Great for a sunny slope. Beautiful red fall color (2 to 3 feet tall).

Hay-scented fern (*Dennstaedtia punctilobula*) Good for shade.

New York fern (*Thelypteris noveboracensis*) Good for shade.

Obedient plant (*Physostegia virginiana*) Spreads into huge colonies that produce magenta flowers in late summer.

St. John's wort (*Hypericum prolificum*) Bright yellow flowers with many medicinal uses. Loves a sunny, dry spot.

All plants listed are North American natives.

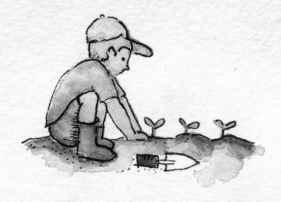

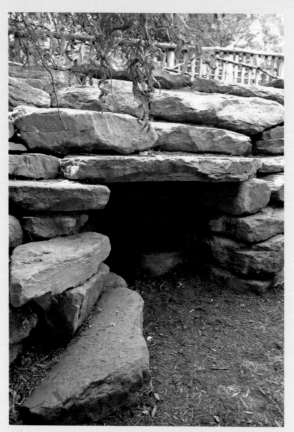

This cave made of large stacked stones is a cozy niche within a hill.

Caves and tunnels

Slopes and hills can also be enhanced by having places to go in, under, and through. A cave can be made of carefully placed stones or timbers inset into the slope, providing that sense of enclosure children seek. If the cave is partway up the slope, it provides a protected perch with a view, which satisfies deep evolutionary drives for simultaneous safety and control over one's territory.

An easy way to create a tunnel through a hill is to use a corrugated drain pipe in as large a diameter as you can find. These are designed to run under roadways and support the weight of vehicles, which makes them sturdy and worry free for play spaces. Tunnels and caves allow different motor skill experiences, such as climbing down into a cave or crawling through a tunnel. Entering a tunnel in one part of the space and exiting in a different place (on the other side of the hill) is an experience that challenges and expands children's understanding of space.

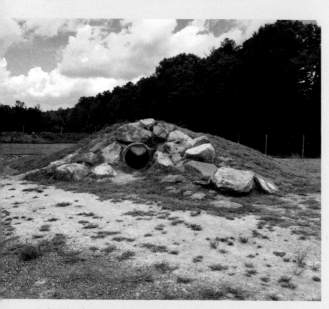

A tunnel passes through this constructed boulder hill.

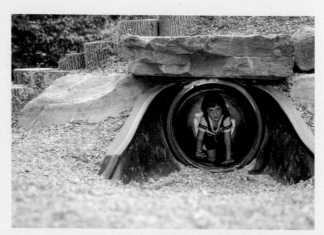

A corrugated drain pipe through a hill is a relatively simple way to create a tunnel. The end is topped with boulders for added variety.

TREES

If you're lucky enough to have good climbing trees in your space, you have the best, most memorable kind of natural climbing. Climbing trees is a primal adventure, a rite of passage, and a challenge that builds strength and confidence. Different kinds of trees require different ways of climbing: up, down, and sideways on gnarly, bouncing, horizontal, and vertical branches. Up in a tree, children often have an expansive view, from a "secret," enclosed, protected vantage point.

Children also may be less likely to injure themselves climbing trees than on playground equipment. One theory is that unlike manufactured equipment, tree branches are uneven in diameter and spacing. The unpredictability of climbing on natural materials requires focused attention that encourages good decision-making as kids navigate up and down. This focus may help keep children safe. To make tree climbing safer, you can remove cracked or weak branches and sharp, protruding points by clipping, lopping, or sawing them off, then sanding. Look for entrapments where small bodies could get stuck and prune the offending areas.

Think about the surfacing below a climbing tree. Soft wood chips are good for the child and the tree: they help cushion falls, and they keep soil aerated, combat soil compaction, and hold in moisture for tree roots. All sorts, shapes, and sizes of trees can be climbed, and they are all valuable learning experiences as children figure out what their bodies can do and test themselves in new ways.

A good climbing tree has somewhat horizontal branches that are low enough to reach and strong enough to support the weight of the climber. Once up in a tree, the view and the sense of being enclosed by greenery provide a uniquely secure and magical perspective for overseeing and understanding the world.

Every tree has its own growing pattern, but if you're planting a tree that you hope will be good for climbing, the accompanying list offers some excellent recommendations. Planting is also an investment in the development of future generations of tree climbers!

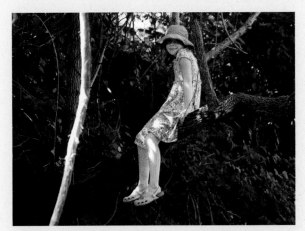

The reward of this climb is perching on a comfy branch.

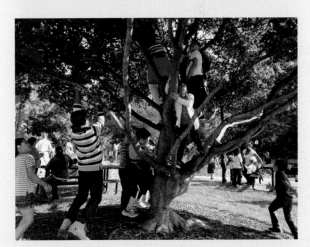

A tree with room for the whole gang to explore, navigate, and hang.

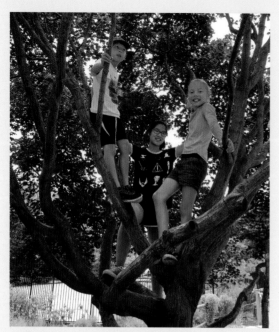

Open branching, such as with this Japanese maple, makes for perfect climbing.

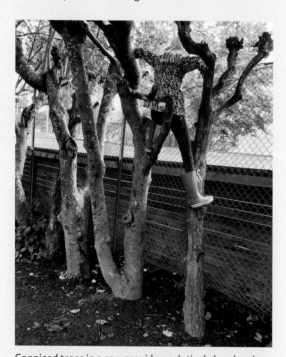

Coppiced trees in a row provide a relatively level series of footholds. (Coppicing is a method of pruning that cuts branches at a certain level and encourages new shoots.) Kids start at one end and move through the branches to the other end without touching the ground.

Great Trees for Climbing

SMALL TREES

Apple* (*Malus pumila*)

Dogwood (*Cornus florida*)

Redbud (*Cercis canadensis*)

LARGE TREES

American beech (*Fagus grandifolia*) Slow growing and strong.

Birch (*Betula* species) Flexible branches make climbing a different experience, but because the branches are often clumping, one can brace oneself and shimmy up.

Elm (*Ulnus* species)

Maple (*Acer* species)

Oak (*Quercus* species) Live oak is wonderful if you live where they can grow; also good for climbing are post oak (*Quercus stellata*), red oak (*Quercus rubra*), and the giant of them all, white oak (*Quercus alba*).

Southern magnolia (*Magnolia grandiflora*) Expect sprawling horizontal branches.

*Indicates non-native. All other plants listed are North American natives.

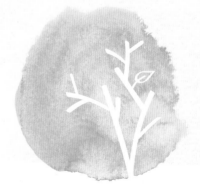

Tree parts

When a tree falls, the silver lining may be the opportunity it offers for kids to scramble onto the trunk and check out the view. Losing a tree that once towered over a garden can be a sad experience, but there is something thrilling about balancing along the length of the trunk and being able to enter the mysterious world of branches that used to be high above.

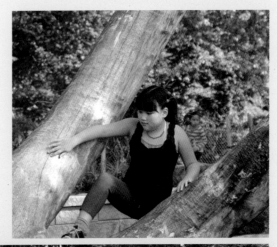

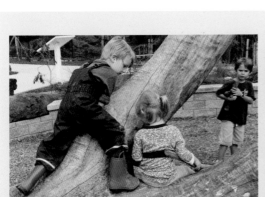

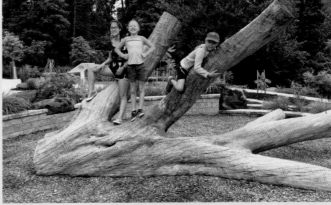

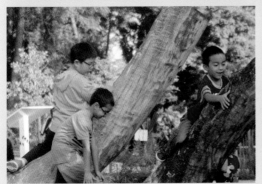

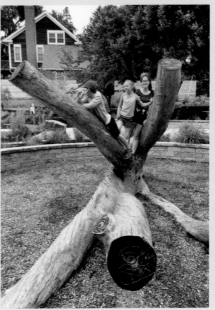

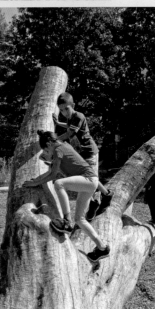

The fallen tree lets kids use their bodies in all sorts of ways. A tree doesn't have to topple in your yard for you to provide the powerful experience of climbing. Installing part of a downed tree or even some logs in your play space offers a natural activity similar to climbing a living tree. An obstacle course on a long serpentine log can offer graded challenges, so kids of different ages, skills, and confidence levels can cross in whatever way they feel comfortable.

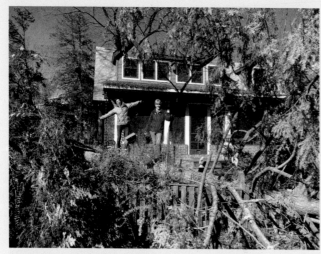

This yard was transformed when a hemlock came down in a windstorm. For a brief while, the front yard became a climbing scape.

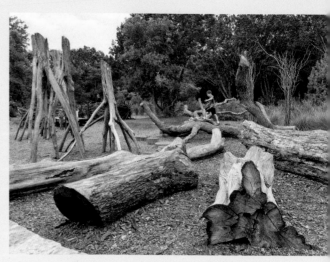

In this nature play area, many logs are laid out to create a challenging, movement-oriented play space.

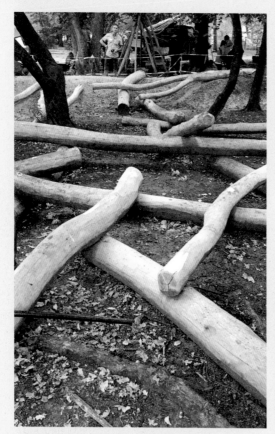

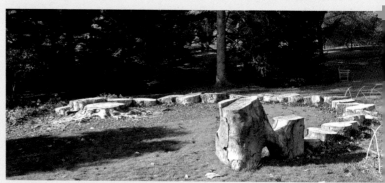

Graduated stumps cut from a downed tree were arranged in an arc curving out from the stump. This artful arrangement creates a path and tells a story of the tree that once grew here.

At the Otto Wels School in Berlin, Germany, a play area features logs arranged like pick-up sticks, though they are securely anchored. The logs define all sorts of spaces for hunkering down and hanging out, and create a multi-path obstacle course for balancing, running, and leaping.

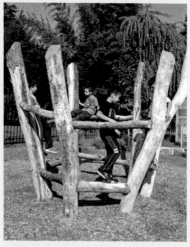

Irregular branches for hanging and sitting develop upper body strength.

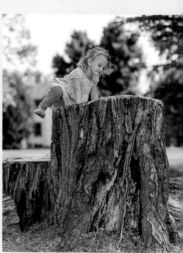

It's a big stretch to get onto this tall stump that was cut and left on the site

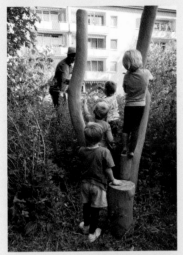

The stilt walk at Löwenzahn Kindergarten in Berlin is designed for whole-body stretching and balancing up off the ground.

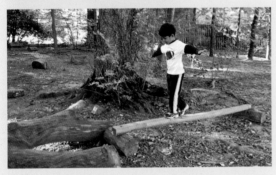

Balancing on a beam set up in the woods.

Using tree parts for play can be a relatively economical way to bring a lot of natural materials and variety into your space: straight, gnarly, or branching logs each invite unique kinds of play. They can be set vertically into the ground or can be laid on top of the ground. Logs with a lot of character will inspire imagination and creative play. If there is potential for a log to shift when many children climb on it, consider stabilizing it with a footer, or more simply, with countersunk spikes driven through the log and into the ground.

If you're not lucky enough to have a tree taken down on your property, you'll need to find branches and parts elsewhere and transport them to your site—a local arborist or tree company may be your best bet. Or, if a tree is coming down in your neighborhood, you may be able to convince the crew to bring some sections to your site. If you do wind up needing to transport the pieces, or to place them in a specific location, equipment such as a tractor or loader or even a crane may be required.

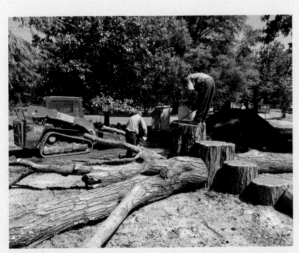

Arranging the pieces of this downed tree includes creating stump steps for climbing and logs positioned for balancing and jumping.

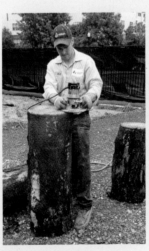

Rounding log edges with a router makes them look more finished and feel more comfortable to sit on.

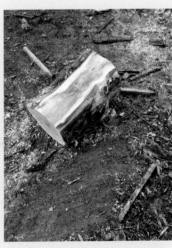

The space between bark and wood holds moisture and provides habitat for damaging insects. Stripping bark extends the life of logs.

ARRANGING TREE PARTS FOR CLIMBING

WHAT YOU'LL NEED

* large sections of downed trees, preferably with parts of trunk and main branches intact
* saw
* shovel
* coarse gravel
* rebar (if necessary)
* wood plugs and glue
* chisel or sander
* router and round-over bit
* wood chips

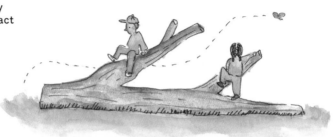

1 Be sure the wood is a long-lasting species, so that it's worth the effort. Black locust (*Robinia pseudoacacia*) is extremely durable; an excellent option for a number of uses in natural play spaces. Eastern red cedar (*Juniperus virginiana*), western red cedar (*Thuja plicata*) and redwood (*Sequoia* species) are rot- and insect-resistant and all are great (and fragrant) choices. Other good options are oak and maple, because both are hardwoods.

2 Choose pieces that are as large as you can accommodate, taking into consideration the size of your play space, access to the final location, and how you're going to move the parts. If you connect with the owner or arborist before the tree is removed, you may be able to specify the parts you want and have them cut accordingly. If possible, cut just below and above the spot where large, sturdy limbs fork. This branching section can be inverted to form an arch or laid on its side to make an interesting climber with multiple paths and levels.

Logs are good, too; the bigger the better for clambering up and jumping off. Big stumps can have a lot of play value as well.

3 Decomposition is a normal part of the life of wood, so it can be a fascinating learning opportunity. You can observe it, discuss it, and document the process with measurements, photos, and drawings. However, if you're going to put some effort into moving a large tree part into place, you'll want to do everything you can to protect the wood. Consider removing the bark. This will help keep the parts dry and insect free, because bark holds moisture against the wood, and provides a home for wood-eating insects. Bark can be stripped with a number of tools: a bark spud, a sharpened straight spade or ice chopper, a draw saw, a chisel, or with a

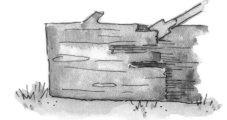

special add-on to your chain saw that works like a planer. You can use any wood sealant rated for outdoor use, but it may be detrimental to seal freshly cut logs, because they will have moisture *inside* that needs to be able to evaporate *out*.

4 Be sure the wood parts won't be sitting in water when it rains. This means digging out the area where they will live and installing 6 to 12 inches of coarse gravel as a bed for the pieces to sit on. This helps rainwater drain away.

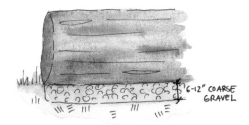

6-12" COARSE GRAVEL

5 All pieces must be anchored securely so they won't shift when children are playing on them. Orient a large fallen tree so it is as stable as possible, even when a whole gang of children is perching on one limb. If needed, stabilize pieces by driving sections of rebar through the wood, countersinking the rebar below the wood surface and covering the depressions with wood plugs.

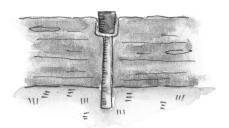

6 Smooth the log to remove any dangerous protrusions or parts that could splinter or poke. Use a saw, chisel, or sander for this.

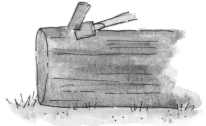

7 Finish cut edges with a router and a round-over bit.

8 Spread a layer of wood chips around the tree parts and 6 feet out in all directions, so that jumping or falling children have a soft place to land. The recommended depth varies with the height that a child could fall, but if the fall height is less than 48 inches, wood chips should be 9 inches deep (which will compact down to 6 inches). For climbing surfaces up to 8 feet high, use 12 inches of wood chips (which will compact down to 9 inches).

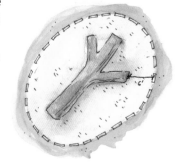

9 Be sure to inspect tree parts regularly. Look for cracks, sharp protrusions, and rotting spots.

See Consumer Product Safety Commission for more detailed information, cpsc.gov.

SWINGS

The experience of moving through space not of your own volition develops the vestibular sense. This sense is based in the inner ear and, as mentioned, is related to balance. A well-developed vestibular sense helps us to understand where our body is in space. Experiences that develop the vestibular sense include swinging, swaying, bouncing, rocking, and rolling. Many yard or play elements support these sorts of movement: bench swings, hammocks, hanging chairs, belt swings, fabric swings, rope swings, tire swings, sensory swings, cradles, baby swings, and more.

THE RISKS OF ELIMINATING RISKS

It can be scary to see your child doing something that seems dangerous. However, it is important for parents to realize that kids need opportunities to make choices, take risks, and do things that are challenging and exciting in order to grow into resilient human beings. Having active-play elements in a natural play space communicates to children that we trust them and want them to get to know themselves, to develop confidence in their abilities, and to learn to make good decisions.

As we build adventure into the design of an outdoor space, we give our children the chance to confront and master their fears and to build self-confidence and self-sufficiency. When children confront risk together, they learn to cooperate and develop empathy and caring. The opposite is also true, as a study from Denmark

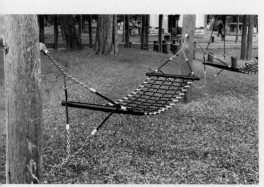

These hammocks have anchor hooks and rope to prevent flipping.

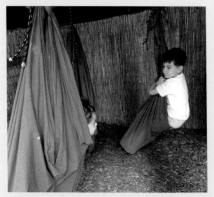

Fabric hung from hooks in the space below a deck provides enveloping softness, soothing motion, and the option to swing and rock in many different positions.

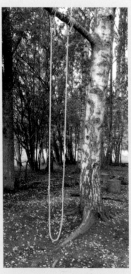

A simple rope loop from a branch is an easily improvised place to swing, standing or sitting.

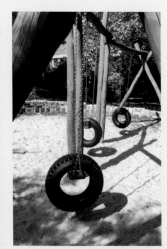

Tire swings can be mounted in different ways for swinging and spinning. Translucent green stain and etchings into the wood make these locust posts extra charming.

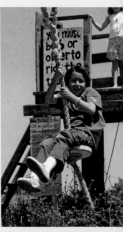

The heavy rope and wooden disc seat of the zipline at the Berkeley Adventure Playground in Berkeley, California, lets kids leap off a raised platform for a thrilling ride.

demonstrates. Children who *don't* have the opportunity to participate in adventurous, somewhat risky play may become irrationally fearful and anxious. They may grow up to be less creative and lack confidence.

Our ancestors took risks, learned from their failures and successes, and survived to bring us into the world. There are some things that cannot be taught, only learned through direct experience. Children are motivated by evolutionary drives to challenge themselves and test their limits.

Children who don't experience the learning that comes from playing in physically challenging spaces may grow up more prone to accidents as adults.

What is acceptable risk? It is important to think about what is required for a child to manage and overcome risk, and this varies with age and experience. This is sometimes described as the difference between a hazard and a risk. A hazard is a danger a child cannot see or understand, versus a risk, which can be seen and understood. It is important, especially if younger children will be using the space, that adults check on the play space and remove hazards.

In determining whether a risk is developmentally appropriate, consider the following components. The child must first be able to recognize a risk: "Wow, there's a big hole in the ground!" The child must then understand the risk: "If I keep running, I'm going to run right into the hole." And finally, they must react to the risk: "I can leap and prepare myself to land in the hole."

Even then, there is a risk of injury. Some consider that if the injury is one that very rarely happens, or is one that a child would be able to heal easily from, then the risk is acceptable.

Risk is everywhere. There is a risk of injury even walking along paved sidewalks. In a natural setting with trees to climb, pointy sticks, slippery rocks, and unexpected holes in the ground, we worry that "something might happen." Instead, the scrapes children acquire should be acknowledged proudly as proof that "you tried to *do* something." At its most basic level, pain is a signal from the environment that leads children to learn how to keep themselves safe. Each bump and bruise is a step in developing resilience. It is through play that children should have the opportunity to test themselves and learn to respond to the environment.

Consider that statistics show that traffic calming (speed bumps and other methods for slowing cars) is ten times more cost effective at saving children's lives than is limiting play. Allowing a child to cross the street alone is a real risk, yet all parents must eventually allow it because they understand it's necessary. The job of parents, teachers, and caregivers is not to succumb to every worry, nor to put their anxiety ahead of what is good for children. Parents need to say yes to outdoor play: yes to running, climbing, getting dirty, and staying outside longer, all in order for our children to grow up with healthy bodies and brains. Sometimes parents just need to sit on their hands, look away, and let children try it.

If you are still concerned about the potential for injury, the International School Grounds Alliance (ISGA) has created the *Risk in Play and Learning Declaration*. It states that play spaces should be "as safe as necessary, not as safe as possible." This may be helpful in weighing the hazards versus the risks in your space. It can be found at internationalschoolgrounds.org/risk/.

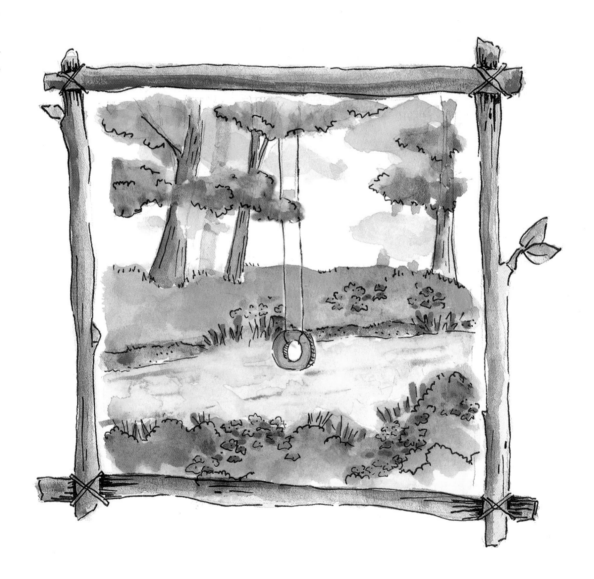

INVITING NATURE

"How does one plan for curiosity, initiative, persistence, risk taking, and resilience? Learning (in nature) often occurs without being taught and without the direct intervention of an adult."

—from *Lens on Outdoor Learning,*
by Wendy Banning and Ginny Sullivan

Natural play and learning spaces celebrate the many dimensions of nature: insects, animals, plants, rocks and minerals, the water cycle, and the cycles of seasons, weather, and life. It's possible to incorporate elements of each of these into your outdoor space in order to draw children's attention to nature, even in a small space. There is much to do and discover outdoors, but a key benefit of connecting to nature may be how it quiets busy little brains.

Time in nature is soothing and healing. A series of studies over the past decade confirms what we know in our hearts: that time in nature clears our heads. Researchers found that the symptoms of children diagnosed with attention deficit disorder were reduced when those children spent time in green spaces (not playing basketball on a paved court, but in nature with quivering leaves and soft breezes). When those children came back indoors, they were more attentive and more cooperative. This applies to everyone. The state of mind we assume when out in nature, sometimes called a state of fascination or reverie, lets our minds wander freely. Known as Attention Restoration Theory, the idea is that time in nature rests the part of our brains required for extensive periods of focused attention in a way that might be as important to our brains as sleep. Don't underestimate the value of taking a walk, pausing on the porch, or spending time in a garden.

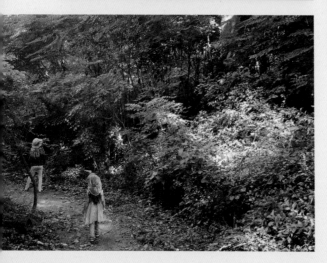

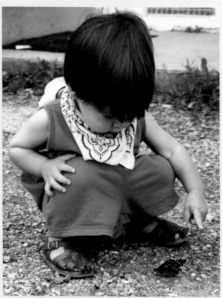

The state of fascination and free-flowing thought that comes most readily in the out-of-doors lets the focused-attention function of our brains rest. This is one reason time in nature reduces stress.

The restorative power of nature is something humans have known throughout history. In the 1800s, patients were sent to sanatoriums in the mountains to recover their health. Research in the 1980s by Robert Ulrich showed that simply having a view of nature healed people. Hospital patients with a view out their window to a green space recovered more quickly and experienced less pain and fewer complications than their counterparts with no access to greenery. Park Rx America is a project that began around 2014 in Washington, DC, and is spreading across the country. In it, doctors are *prescribing* time in nature—such as walks through parks on the way to school—and seeing dramatic results in mood and physical health. The book *Shinrin Yoku: The Japanese Art of Forest Bathing* (2018) describes a time-honored practice which began in the old-growth forests of Japan and has arrived in the United States. It cites research that shows people who spend time outside among trees are less depressed and less susceptible to disease. All of this comes under the umbrella of the burgeoning field of ecotherapy. Nature heals us.

SURROUNDING CHILDREN WITH INTRIGUING PLANTS

For me, plants are the heart of the design palette in natural play and learning spaces, and deserve a special focus. Plants define spaces. They can be arranged to create an edge (a hedge of native shrubs with varied bark, berries, flowers, and fall leaf colors), an enclosure (grasses and boulders surrounding a secret niche), a soft carpet (pine needles), or a fragrant ceiling (wisteria). Plants add texture to a space—from the softness of lamb's ears or Mexican feather grass, to

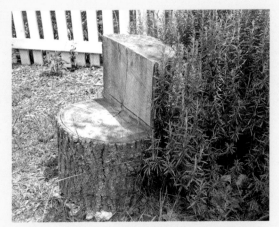

The aroma of rosemary greets those who rest at this stump seat.

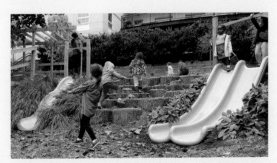

Lamb's ears and Mexican feather grass on the hill beside slides add softness when children brush up against the plants.

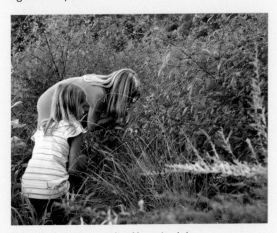

Grasses thrive in a wetland learning lab.

the smooth bark of a beech tree, to the explosive surprise of a popping jewelweed seed pod. There is no end to the value of plants as basic ingredients of a children's play space: the colors, the way they filter light, the fragrance, and the pickable loose parts.

Plants are much more than design elements, however. Ponder with your children how essential plants are to our lives in so many ways. Plants are food, and if we eat further up the food chain, plants are the food for our food. There is pretty much nothing we eat, except maybe minerals like salt and iron and zinc, that doesn't come from or depend on plants. Without plants (and the insects that pollinate many of them), there would be no food for any creature, humans included. Without plants, there would be no furniture or houses or any kind of shelter built of wood. Without plants to exhale the very oxygen we need to survive, there would be no life on our planet. Plants bring color, texture, fragrance, food, shelter, and softness to the world. Our children's connection to them in our outdoor spaces is fundamental.

One interesting bit of research cited in *Last Child in the Woods* compares social hierarchies within groups of children and how that changes, based on the environments where the kids play. When children played in an outdoor environment dominated by commercially produced play structures, the leaders tended to be the strongest and most athletic. Playing in an area with plants and loose parts, the leaders were the most creative, inventive, and verbal kids. Having such children as leaders and peer role models exposes all children to creative thinking

and verbal rather than physical negotiating and problem-solving. Nature helps us get along.

Going native

Native plants create a connection to place and a sense of local identity. The birches, firs, and maples of the Northeast, the aspens and spruces of the Rockies, the redwoods of the Pacific Northwest, and the magnolias, loblollies, and live oaks of the South—each creates a unique sense of place that without words tells us where we are. Children deserve to be surrounded by uniquely local plants so that they grow up securely rooted to home. Many native plants have unique qualities in terms of color, fragrance, and texture. Plant as many as you have space for, to give kids exposure to their variety and wonder.

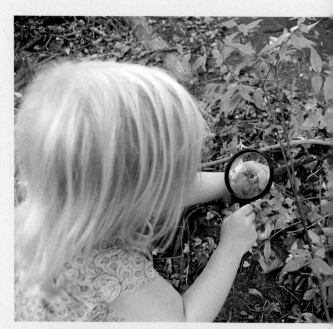

Euonymus americanus in bloom has a colorful red seed pod with orange berries inside. Definitely worth close examination.

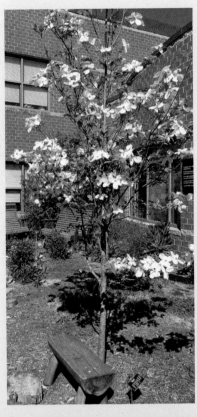

Spring-blooming dogwood is a compact tree for sunny or understory spots.

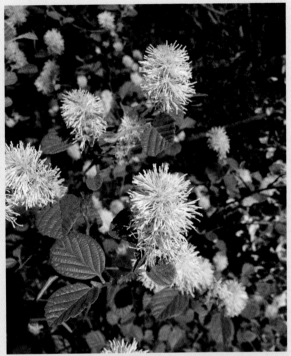

Fothergilla has honey-scented, pom-pom-shaped blooms in early spring and bright orange fall foliage that make it appealing to kids in both seasons.

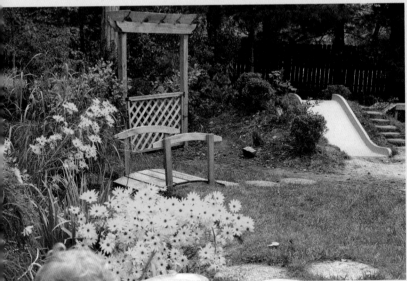

Ox-eye sunflower in bloom is a riot of sunny brightness; abundant flowers invite picking.

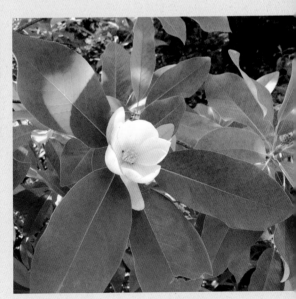

Lemon-scented sweet bay magnolia is a large, semievergreen tree with interesting seed pods in the fall.

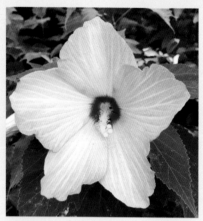

This hibiscus flower is almost 12 inches in diameter on a plant that can be about 3 feet tall.

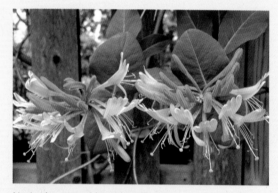

Native honeysuckle adds color along an entry fence. The native species is sadly not as fragrant as the invasive variety, but is better for the ecosystem, as it attracts pollinating insects and hummingbirds.

Native plants are well adapted to the local climate and soil. They are the foundation of our ecosystem because they provide the best and sometimes only food for our wildlife. Having evolved alongside local insects and animals, native plants are an essential and digestible source of food for these creatures. According to Doug Tallamy, author of *Bringing Nature Home*, if you want to invite songbirds to your yard, plant native plants. Professor Tallamy tells us that a clutch of baby chickadees needs to eat 390 to 570 caterpillars *each day* for the 16 to18 days it takes them to reach maturity. Planting native plants in your yard brings the native insects who eat them. Mama birds will be likely to nest near a backyard that provides an abundance of the food their babies need. It's exciting for the whole family to have a nest in the yard, hopefully with hatching eggs and baby birds to watch. Why not provide ecosystem services as you provide play space for your children?

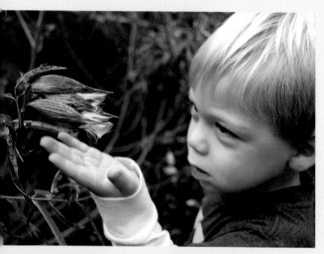

The soft down inside a milkweed pod in autumn is irresistible to touch.

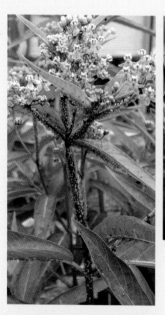

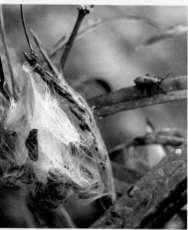

Swamp milkweed hosting lots of aphids (left), and in the late summer with milkweed beetles (right).

IDENTIFYING NATIVE MILKWEED

Native milkweed is food for monarch butterflies. According to the National Wildlife Federation, there are twelve species of milkweed that are native to different regions of North America, and those are the *only* species homeowners should plant. The twelve are: swamp milkweed (*Asclepias incarnata*), common milkweed (*Asclepias syriaca*), butterfly weed (*Asclepias tuberosa*), spider milkweed (*Asclepias asperula*) purple milkweed (*Asclepias purpurascens*), showy milkweed (*Asclepias speciosa*), California milkweed (*Asclepias californica*), white milkweed (*Asclepias variegata*), whorled milkweed (*Asclepias verticillata*), Mexican whorled milkweed (*Asclepias fascicularis*), desert milkweed (*Asclepias erosa*), and green milkweed (*Asclepias viridis*).

Late in the season, fluffy seeds burst out of the milkweed pods and provide a magical play material for children.

Some insects, caterpillars especially, can only eat one food; others are less choosy. Native plants will attract an array of interesting insects to your garden. Early exposure to the important role of native plants as habitat lays the groundwork for children to be environmental stewards.

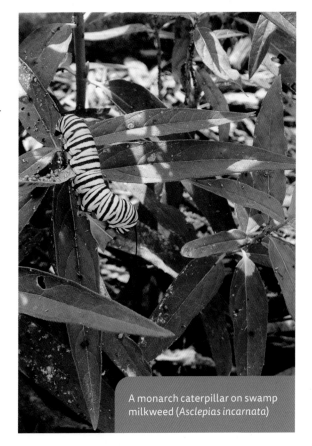

A monarch caterpillar on swamp milkweed (*Asclepias incarnata*)

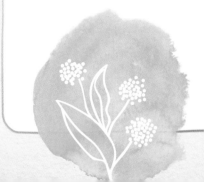

The accompanying plant list was originally created for the Reading Garden at Drew Model Elementary School in Virginia. The list includes trees, shrubs, vines, grasses, and perennials that bring four seasons of color and lots of wildlife value to a courtyard garden. We added to the literacy value of the garden with custom-made Smart Garden ABCs garden signs (smartgarden-signs.com). These show botanical and common names, with the first letter of the common name highlighted, plus facts about the plant and its medicinal, food, or wildlife value.

AN ALPHABET of NATIVE PLANTS

LETTER	COMMON NAME	BOTANICAL NAME
A	aster	*Symphyotrichum novae-angliae*
B	beebalm	*Monarda didyma*
C	cardinal flower	*Lobelia cardinalis*
D	dogwood	*Cornus florida*
E	echinacea (also coneflower)	*Echinacea purpurea*
F	fringetree	*Chionanthus virginicus*
G	goldenrod	*Solidago 'Goldstrahl'*
H	hibiscus	*Hibiscus 'Lord Baltimore'*
I	iris	*Iris versicolor*
J	Jacob's-ladder	*Polemonium foliosissimum*
K	kinnikinnick	*Arctostaphylos uva-ursi*
L	love grass	*Eragrostis spectabilis*
M	milkweed	*Asclepias tuberosa*
N	nassella (also feather grass)	*Nassella tenuissima*
O	obedient plant	*Physostegia virginiana*
P	pink	*Silene caroliniana*

LETTER	COMMON NAME	BOTANICAL NAME
Q	quercus (also red oak)	*Quercus rubra*
R	red twig dogwood	*Cornus sericea*
S	serviceberry	*Amelanchier χ grandiflora*
T	trumpet vine	*Campsis radicans*
U	uvularia (also bellwort)	*Uvularia perfoliata*
V	violet	*Viola labradorica*
W	winterberry	*Ilex verticillata*
X	xanthorhiza (also yellowroot)	*Xanthorhiza simplicissima*
Y	yucca	*Yucca filamentosa*
Z	zizia	*Zizia aurea*

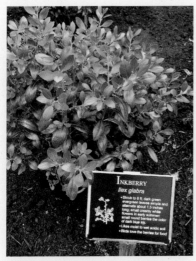

If you're involved with your child's school garden or a local pocket park, consider encouraging the use of Smart Garden signs. These plant identification plaques teach children plant facts.

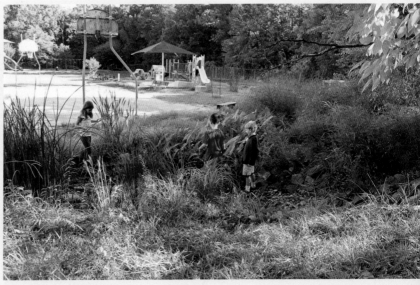

Use the perimeter of the play space to add interesting, colorful, and educational nature areas. A small wetland planting adjacent to a schoolyard makes the site more inviting for kids and wildlife alike.

Invasive plants

Each state has a list of plants considered invasive. Invasive plants are those that did not evolve in an area, but were brought in (either intentionally or accidentally) and escaped into the wild, where they occupy habitat, crowd out native plants, and cause harm to the environment. Of the woody plants considered invasive, 85 percent escaped into wild spaces from gardens. The site Invasive-PlantAtlas.org is a very helpful source of information organized by region, and there are many others resources available online. The difference in whether a plant is considered invasive or not is often merely a question of where it grows. Many invasives were brought to places because they had some quality people valued—perhaps beautiful fall color (burning bush and nandina), pretty spring flowers and a tendency to grow quickly (Bradford pear and Chinese wisteria), or a root system that prevents erosion (English ivy and kudzu).

In nature, all human disruptions have consequences. It was an unintended consequence that these plants escaped into the wild and began to cause harm. Take English ivy, for example. Birds eat the berries of the ivy, poop them out in the forests, where seeds sprout, roots take hold, and the wandering stems strangle trees and smother neighboring plants. Chinese wisteria, burning bush, and Bradford pear fill wild spaces with their offspring, crowding out the native plants our wildlife needs. Cedar waxwings are drawn to the bright red berries of nandina, but are poisoned by toxins in those berries. Some imported plants can be well-behaved in the garden for years, until a subtle change causes them to suddenly start popping up in the wild.

At this point, it is generally not illegal for nurseries to sell invasive plants, so it is not illegal to purchase them (although in my opinion both selling and purchasing should be). However, it can be catastrophic to the environment to plant or grow these invasive species—so please don't! There are many, many native alternatives, as well as a few non-native-but-not-invasive special plants, that I recommend throughout this book. Another caution, though: shop carefully. In an ironic twist, many nursery plants, natives included, are treated with neonicotinoids, which have been known to kill honeybees and contribute to the phenomenon of colony collapse.

Protecting kids from plants

Most plants bring only good into children's lives, but there are a few cautions when including plants in a play space. Despite the colorful berries on evergreen hollies, I don't recommend them or any plant with prickly leaves for a garden that

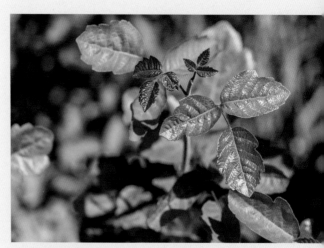

Poison oak is most common in West Coast states, growing as a small shrub. Its hallmark is its leaves, which grow in sets of three, with wavy or scalloped edges and rounded tips. The leaves may or may not be shiny.

welcomes children. Running barefoot is such an important part of being a wild child and pointy holly leaves on the ground don't mix well with small, defenseless feet. In that same vein, I recommend avoiding or even removing plants with lots of thorns, such as hawthorn (*Crataegus*) or devil's walking stick (*Aralia spinosa*), and grasses with razor-sharp leaf edges such as non-native pampas grass. It's important for children to learn to recognize poison ivy and poison oak, so I commend places like the North Carolina Botanical Garden for maintaining a poison garden with such plants growing and labeled. However, these plants clearly don't belong in a place where children are meant to wander freely, so it's important to remove such nuisances, whether by pulling them out by the roots (be sure to wear protective gloves and gear to cover all exposed skin), or by careful spraying. If an irritating plant is unknowingly encountered and causes a skin rash, there are natural remedies such as jewelweed

(*Impatiens capensis*) and plantain (*Plantago major*) that can be applied. Rub the sap from stems and leaves of either plant on newly exposed skin, or make a tea with jewelweed to bathe in or freeze for soothing ice cubes.

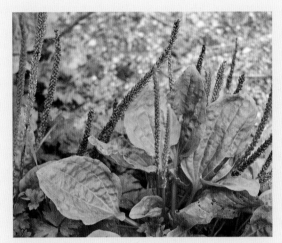

Sometimes known as nature's Band-Aid, plantain heals cuts and scrapes. Rub a leaf on skin exposed to irritating plants to help soothe pain and itchy skin rashes.

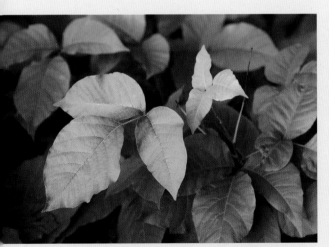

Poison ivy is more common in the East and Midwest. It too has leaves that appear in threes and may or may not be shiny. Poison ivy generally grows as a vine, and the tips of its leaves are usually pointed.

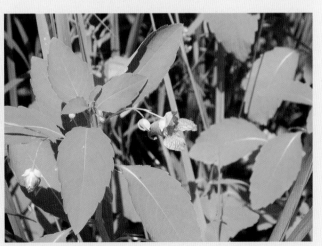

The sap of jewelweed can counter the effects of poison ivy and poison oak. Rub it on the affected skin after being exposed. Jewelweed is also known as touch-me-not. Kids love the ripe seed pods, because they pop with great drama when lightly touched.

In my view, it is important to understand and make informed decisions about plants considered poisonous because there are varying degrees of toxicity. Try to make sound choices by weighing the degree of risk against any potential benefit of including a plant in your space. Some, such as iris, are considered mildly toxic because their roots can cause an upset tummy for a short period of time if consumed by the bushel. Others, such as pokeweed (*Phytolacca americana*) and Carolina jessamine (*Gelsemium sempervirens*), are so poisonous that ingesting just one leaf of jessamine or one berry of pokeweed can bring tragic consequences. The abundant yellow flowers that cover Carolina jessamine look like honeysuckle. That could fool a child who knows the trick of getting one drop of sweet nectar from a honeysuckle blossom. Never plant this in a garden where children will play. Understanding that some plants are mildly toxic (the leaves

of tomatoes, the bulbs of daffodils, for example) but still offer valuable benefits may allow you to decide that in your garden, the benefits outweigh the risks. A great website that lists plants and describes their toxicity is https://plants.ces.ncsu.edu/plants/category/poisonous-plants/.

Protecting plants from kids

The reason we have plants in the play space is so children can interact with them as closely as possible. For new plants to successfully establish, though, it is essential to protect them from the traffic of little feet.

The goal is for children to have a clear visual and physical reminder not to step on vulnerable young plants. This can be accomplished in lots of ways. Clearly defined bed edges are a great help. It takes about two years for woody plants to become well established. After that, it's okay to remove the edging and allow children to play

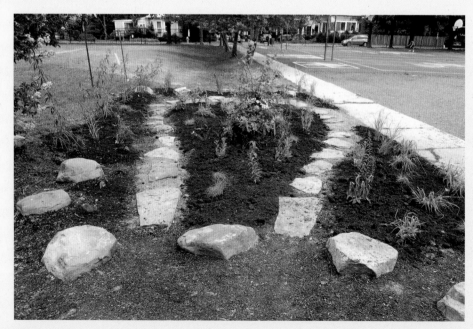

A stone path before (left) and after (right) a pollinator garden grows and fills in.

in and under the shrubs, trees, and woody vines (note that herbaceous perennials will always need some protection). To maintain plants in a group setting, rope them off from foot traffic each year during early spring to protect delicate new shoots.

Use a type of mulch around plants that is clearly different from the mulch used on pathways and play spaces. I recommend leaf mulch (Leaf Gro), which offers all the benefits of a good organic mulch—it holds in moisture, keeps down weeds, and improves the soil as it decomposes. Unlike wood mulch, which is also used in pathways, leaf mulch looks dark and more like soil. It is a visual signal to children that this is a planting bed.

Small borders and edging help to physically keep children from walking in the planted areas. Some edging ideas:

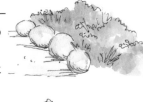

- Medium-sized rocks—too big for children to carry easily, but not large enough to block the view

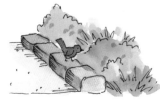

- Wall stones set into the ground on edge
- Cobblestones or bricks

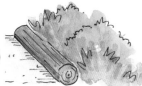

- Logs (3 to 6 inches in diameter is a good size) laid along the ground

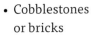

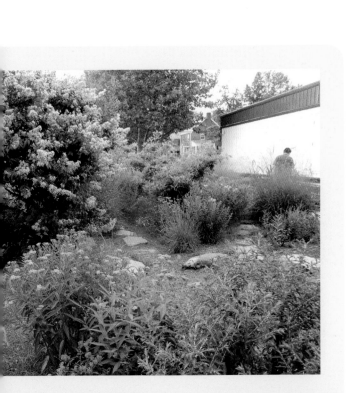

- Posts spaced 6 to 8 inches apart, with a hole drilled in each and rope run between the posts. These can be anywhere from 9 to 24 inches tall; tall enough to notice, not so tall that children can walk under them. Lower is better. Tops can be rounded. Posts can be 4-by-4-inch timbers, rough log posts, metal, or anything similar.

- Wood or composite boards set on edge

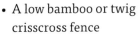

- A low bamboo or twig crisscross fence

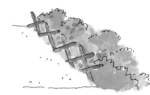

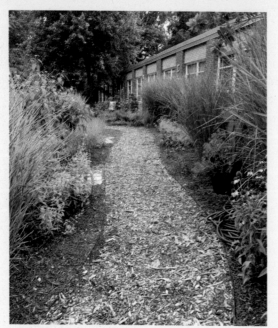

Different kinds of mulch distinguish planting beds from this walking path, which helps protect plants from trampling feet.

CALLING ATTENTION TO NATURAL CYCLES AND MATERIALS

Bark peels off an old stump, puddles shrink and disappear, mushrooms sprout in damp soil, beetles take up residence under a log. Children stay interested in natural spaces because nature is always changing and never boring. The design of a natural play space can highlight natural cycles of time, weather, and life.

Materials such as stone, tree parts, plants, water, and sand bring textural variety to a space and are sustainable because they break down naturally or can easily be reused. We can use tree parts of many sorts and sizes, from milled boards to crooked sticks, from tiny cookies cut from slender branches to a 2-ton fallen tree. These all decompose, which is part of what makes them fascinating, and they are easy to replace, especially if you befriend your local arborist. Stone at a full range of scales can be part of a natural play space, from tiny bits of gravel, to flat flagstone slabs, to giant round boulders. Boulders are so long lasting that Native Americans called them grandmothers; they stay around and bear witness to changes in the more ephemeral aspects of life and nature.

For some planting areas, this edging will need to be permanent, so children can interact with the plants by coming up to the edge of the bed, but not walking in the bed. For other areas, especially those with tough shrubs and grasses, the edging can be removed once the plants are established, allowing kids to play around and under plants. You may want to bring edging back in the spring, to protect emerging new shoots for the first few weeks.

Obvious pathways through planted beds allow children to pass through, but show them exactly where it's okay to step.

Raised beds elevate plants, often to a more convenient level for children to interact, while discouraging foot traffic. Raised beds can be made of all sorts of materials, including logs, boards, timbers, or posts set on end or horizontally.

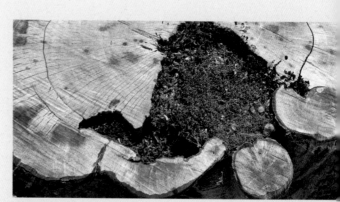

Leave a cut stump in place so children can observe the decomposition over time.

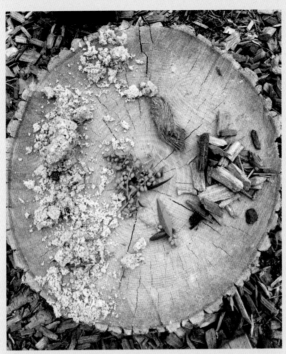

Assorted bits of nature, arranged with care.

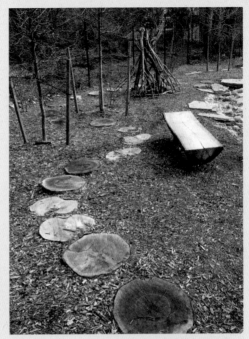

A tree cookie path leads to a split-log bench with a stream and branch hut in the background.

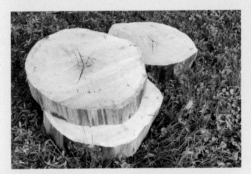

Provide loose tree cookies for play—you'll be amazed at how many different uses children can find for them.

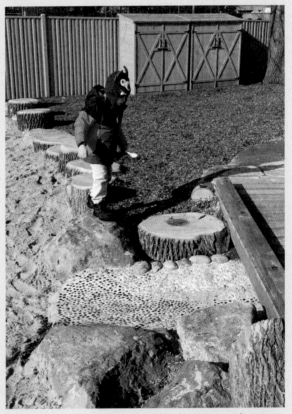

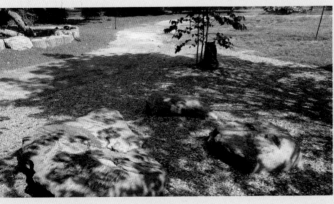

Boulders in dappled shade.

A rich variety of materials—boulders, stumps, sand, stone, and wood chips—in the corner of a play space.

Consider the changing light through a day and across seasons. Planting grasses along the east or west side of your site may allow them to be backlit in the early morning or afternoon when the sun is low in the sky. Notice the patterns of shadows throughout the day and year. Leave buckets out to collect rain and add tools like thermometers and rain gauges to measure changes over time. Weather vanes, whirligigs, flapping flags, and chimes all make the wind visible. Choose plants for spring and summer flowers, but also fall foliage.

The cycles of birth and nourishment, living and growing, dying and decomposition happen over and over in the natural world, on many different levels and scales. Encourage children to

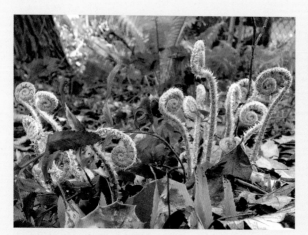

Fiddleheads emerge in spring.

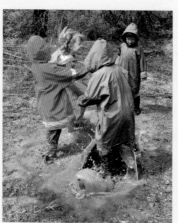

The right gear makes it easy to revel in a rainy April walk.

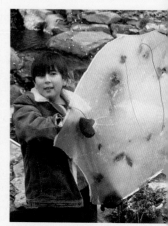

Ice formed on the backyard pond overnight!

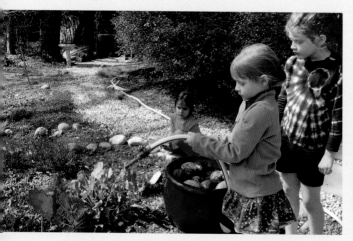

Caring for the garden brings anticipation of a new growing season.

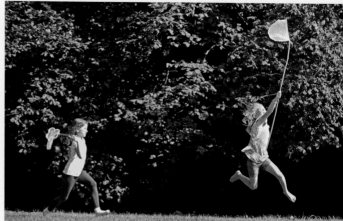

Summer means lots of running barefoot and maybe catching a few bugs.

observe new spring shoots, measure the zucchini in the garden, and watch fledgling birds and caterpillars. Notice and examine rotting logs. When you see a dead bird or beetle, talk about it with your child. Paying attention to the totality of the life cycle prepares children for celebrating life and understanding and grieving death and loss in healthy ways.

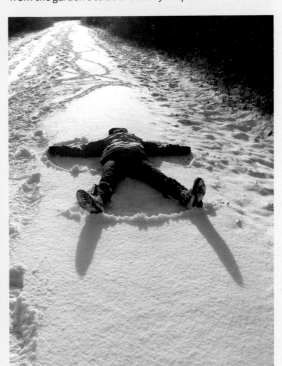

Warm weather fun: enjoying watermelon from the garden beside the backyard pond.

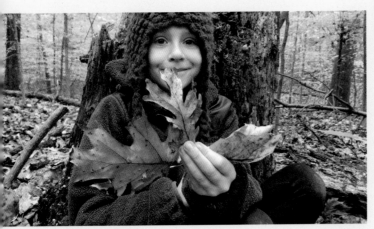

Autumn brings fallen leaves galore.

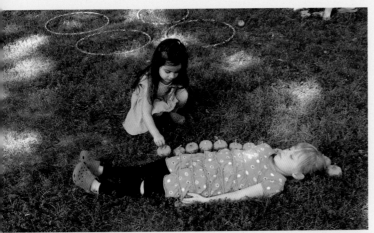

Once harvested in the fall, mini pumpkins inspire all sorts of creative play.

Low light on a winter afternoon illuminates snow play.

Ephemeral Plants for a Spring Surprise

Spring ephemerals are plants that appear, bloom, and die back without a trace early in the growing season, before the heat of summer. Plant these in the fall in a shape—a giant circle, heart, square, or squiggle—that will delight in spring when the blooms appear in the lawn. In a few weeks, they will disappear completely.

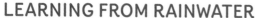

Crested iris (*Iris cristata*) Blue or white flowers

Crocus* (*Crocus* species) White, purple, or blue flowers

Grape hyacinth* (*Muscari* species) Blue, purple, or white fragrant flowers

Snowdrop* (*Galanthus nivalis*) White flowers

Trout lily (*Erythronium americanum*) Yellow flowers

Virginia bluebells (*Mertensia virginica*) Periwinkle blue flowers

Woodland phlox (*Phlox divaricata*) Powder blue flowers

*Indicates non-native. All other plants listed are North American natives.

LEARNING FROM RAINWATER

The old approach to managing stormwater was to quickly send it "away." That usually meant huge quantities of water piped into storm drains, then gushing into our streams at high volumes. This washed away lots of stream bank soil, which caused damaging erosion and carried large quantities of choking sediment to rivers and bays. Professionals (designers, planners, engineers, ecologists) and homeowners are beginning to understand that the best way to manage stormwater is to keep it on-site and let it soak into the ground. This slows, cleans, and cools the water, so that by the time it seeps into streams, it doesn't cause erosion. Cleaner water improves the health of our rivers and bays.

A rain garden is a bowl-shaped planted area designed to capture rainwater and hold it while it soaks into the ground. Having a rain garden in your yard is a great way for children to see the water cycle in action. Direct the roof water from your downspouts to your rain garden and wait for the next rainstorm! It is fascinating to watch your rain garden become a pond during a storm—within hours, the water will soak completely into the ground. Many states and localities have programs to help homeowners build (and even pay for) rain gardens, because these gardens have such a positive impact on the watershed. There may be local guidelines for the best way to build such a garden in your area. Generally, it's good to use a special soil mix that contains lots of sand, and to incorporate plants that are well adapted to both drought and deluge. Native plants in particular offer ecological benefits. Their roots work with the porous soil to absorb and filter stormwater. The plants themselves provide habitat and food for beneficial insects and other wildlife.

To make your rain garden friendly to kids, add a stepping stone path through it (for use on dry days) or a bridge across it (to use anytime). Children can watch the rain garden do its work on rainy days. When the weather is dry, little ones can get up close to the plants and insects happily inhabiting the garden.

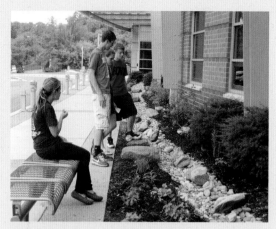

A previously drab entry to this school was transformed by students into a lush bioswale that absorbs rainwater from the glass canopy and adds habitat and beauty to the school entry. The same treatment could be applied to border plantings along the perimeter of any home.

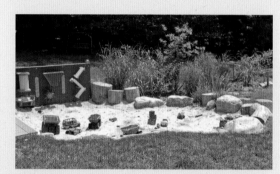

This sand area and the adjacent rain garden capture lots of rainwater.

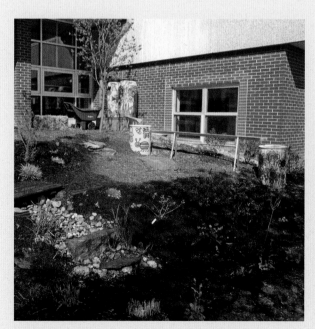

Brightly colored rain barrels catch the downspout water. Overflow goes into dry streams and then into the rain garden.

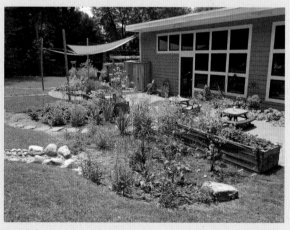

Water from a play stream empties into a rain garden planted with natives.

RAIN GARDEN PLANTS with FUN NAMES

PLANT	DESCRIPTION
TREES	
River birch (*Betula nigra*)	Great textured bark; often grows in clusters of three or more trunks which are very graceful.
Serviceberry (*Amelanchier* species)	White flowers in spring, edible (by birds and humans) berries in early summer, yellow fall color, smooth gray bark. Can be a large shrub or a small tree.
Musclewood (*Carpinus caroliniana*)	Smooth bark on a ribbed trunk. Ribs look like muscles.
SHRUBS	
Buttonbush (*Cephalanthus occidentalis*)	Funny pods that look like little space ships. One variety is even called 'Sputnik'. Pioneers used the pods as buttons.
Red twig dogwood (*Cornus sericea* 'Cardinal')	White flowers in spring, soft yellow fall leaves, beautiful bright red bark in winter. Cut twigs are great for crafts.
Yellow twig dogwood (*Cornus sericea* 'Flaviramea')	White flowers in spring, soft yellow fall leaves, beautiful yellow bark in winter. Cut twigs are great for crafts.
Sweetshrub (*Calycanthus floridus*)	Fragrant burgundy or yellow flowers in late spring. Blooms smell like sour apple.
Winterberry (*Ilex verticillata*)	Females produce bright red berries in fall and winter if you have one male planted somewhere in the vicinity. Berries provide food for birds and color in the garden.
Inkberry (*Ilex glabra*)	The female of this non-prickly, evergreen holly will produce dark blue berries if you have a male nearby.

PLANT	DESCRIPTION
PERENNIALS	
Swamp milkweed (*Asclepias incarnata*)	Pink flowers in early summer provide nectar for beneficial bees and butterflies, but the leaves are the most important part: they are the only food that monarch caterpillars eat.
Turtlehead (*Chelone obliqua*)	Pink flowers beloved by butterflies and hummingbirds.
Blue mist flower (Conoclinium coelestinum)	Gorgeous shade of periwinkle blue flowers that butterflies love. Blooms through summer into fall. Spreads into colonies when it's happy. Likes dry or wet conditions.
Cardinal flower (*Lobelia cardinalis*)	Vertical spikes of bright red flowers. Loves wet soil in partial sun. Hummingbirds can't resist this one!
Rose mallow (*Hibiscus moscheutos*)	Pale pink to magenta flowers the size of dinner plates in mid- to late summer.
Ironweed (*Vernonia noveboracensis*)	Giant stalks (6 feet or more) with magenta flowers. Dwarf variety is called 'Iron Butterfly' which grows to about 3 feet tall.
Joe Pye weed (*Eutrochium purpureum*)	Tall—6 to 8 feet—with pinkish purple flowers beloved by butterflies.

All plants listed are North American natives.

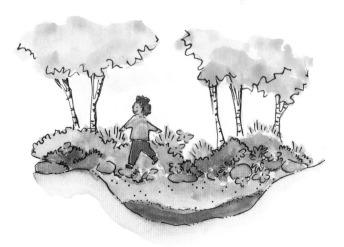

WELCOMING WILDLIFE

Providing habitat is good for the planet and welcoming birds, bugs, toads, and turtles into your yard can be fascinating for your family. To do this, you need to provide the habitat these creatures need. That includes food, shelter, water, and places for wildlife to raise their young.

One of the requirements for attracting wildlife is providing the plants that young and adult insects, birds, and small mammals need to eat, including particular leaves, flowers, and berries. Think about the materials they like to use for shelter, the surfaces where they lay their eggs, and the environments they choose for undergoing metamorphosis. Certain insects winter over inside the hollow stems of dried herbaceous plants, so *don't* cut back grasses and perennials in the fall. If a tree in your yard needs to come down, consider leaving a portion standing. This is called a snag and it can provide rich habitat for insects and birds like woodpeckers.

A backyard birdbath attracts a female Northern Cardinal.

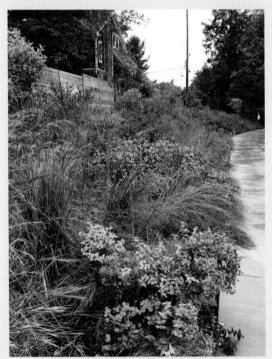

Grasses and perennials offer both food and habitat for wildlife. For more information on making your yard a nature haven, read *Bringing Nature Home*.

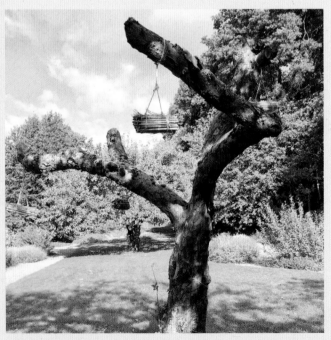

Bundles of hollow twigs are a very simple way to provide habitat.

YARD FEATURES THAT ATTRACT WILDLIFE

BRUSH PILE

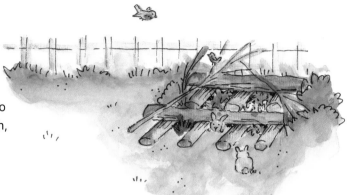

Brush piles provide important shelter for rabbits and other small mammals, reptiles, frogs, and toads, as well as ground birds and insects. It is a place to hide from predators, to nest, to raise young, and to find food, warmth, and cover from the elements.

WHAT YOU'LL NEED

* fallen branches
* logs
* prunings from trees and shrubs

1 Choose a spot in a protected corner of your yard. If you live near woods or water, this is a valuable addition to the edge—where the forest meets a field or land meets water. Make sure the spot is well drained, so the space below the brush pile is dry.

2 Arrange the largest logs (6 to 10 inches in diameter) at the base, parallel to each other, with 6 to 12 inches in between.

3 On top of the base logs, add another row of logs perpendicular to the base logs, creating a multi-level crisscross.

4 Pile branches on top of the logs, larger to smaller as you go up. Leave gaps for air space and hiding places as you pile.

BIRD BLIND

Bird blinds let children get up close to observe and experience birds. Peek through the windows for a close-up look at the avian visitors to your garden enjoying bird-friendly plants, feeders, birdbaths, and birdhouses on the other side.

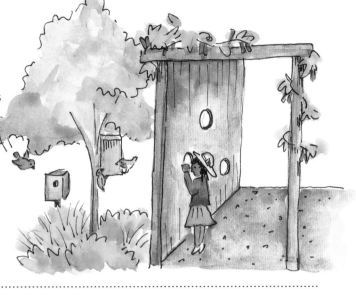

WHAT YOU'LL NEED

* Section(s) of solid fence and any required structural support
* Material for roof, if roof is desired
* Saw for cutting holes

1 Cut peephole windows in the fence section facing the viewing area, at child and adult heights.

2 Add a vine-covered trellis or roof above so that birds can't see human observers.

3 Add bird feeders and bird-friendly plants to the other side.

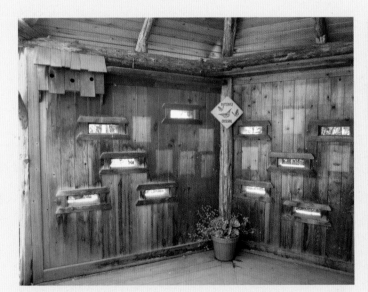

A bird blind with at least two walls and a roof works best.

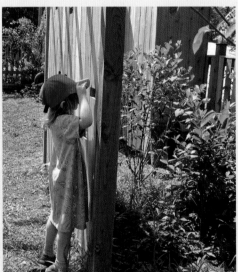

Peeking through at the birds. Note that a blind can be placed in an otherwise unused side yard.

BACKYARD POND

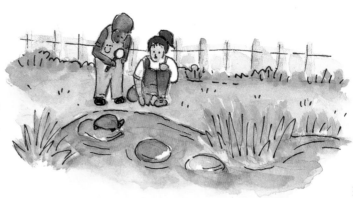

Having a pond in your yard provides drinking water for birds and mammals, as well as a home for dragonflies, frogs, turtles, and fish. There is a fun and beautiful group of water garden plants to grow in your pond (that never need to be watered). With a recirculating pump to keep the water flowing and mosquitoes from breeding, and fish to eat the plant detritus and poop out fertilizer for the plants, a pond doesn't have to be a lot of work. It provides both habitat value and play value—animals and plants to observe, plus a very satisfying place to drop rocks. Helpful DIY instructions for building a backyard pond can be found at empressofdirt.net/build-backyard-pond/ and other gardening websites.

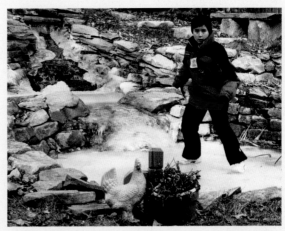

Ponds can offer adventure and learning opportunities even during cold months. In winter, this backyard pond freezes with ice several inches thick.

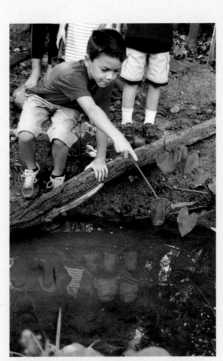

Spotting pond inhabitants and watching their activities can keep children engaged for hours.

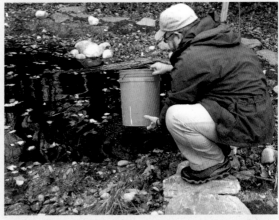

"Seeding" a new backyard pond with muck from a nearby woodland pool introduces microorganisms and macro-invertebrates that will populate the pond and begin to establish a food chain to support frogs and larger creatures.

INSECT HOTEL

Beneficial insects pollinate plants and control the pests who eat our food plants or sting us. An insect hotel is a structure built with natural materials to provide a variety of nesting spots for different types of beneficial insects and small animals. Place your insect hotel in your pollinator garden so that the plants and this habitat house will work together to welcome the critters you want to attract. Your hotel can include a variety of materials to create cavities of different kinds that will attract beneficial insects, and also make the hotel look interesting. Here is one version of an insect hotel that can be an easy weekend project.

INVITING NATURE

134

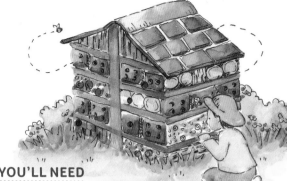

WHAT YOU'LL NEED

* wooden shipping pallets (number to be determined by desired height of structure)
* bricks
* sticks, straw
* hollow stems (examples: bamboo, aster, cup plant, Joe Pye weed)
* pinecones
* rocks
* mud
* cob (soil, sand, straw, water)
* pencil, skewer

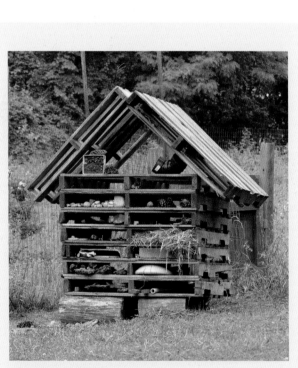

Scavenged supplies and shipping pallets makes this an economical project. Kids can work on every step of the process.

1. (optional) Create a base for pallets to rest on.
2. Stack pallets on base or ground, then on top of each other, to desired height.
3. Stuff openings with a variety of materials, including bricks, pinecones, mud, and other materials from nature. Hollow stems of different diameters are a great addition. If you wish to house bees, cut the hollow pieces at a node so the back of each tunnel is closed (bees won't nest in tunnels that are open at both ends).
4. Cob is a perfect material to make nesting blocks for the hotel. A nesting block is a brick-like cube with tiny tunnels that provide shelter for insects. Mix some soil, sand, and straw with water.
5. Form the cob into a block that is at least 6 inches deep. Poke some holes in it with a pencil, and some with a long skewer.
6. Let the block dry and add it to your hotel.

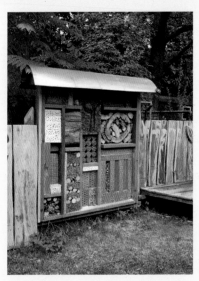

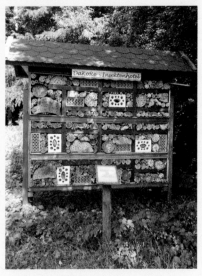

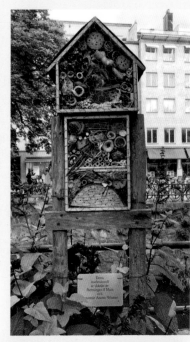

An assortment of inspiring single- and multi-sided insect hotels from around the world (all with important overhangs to protect from rain), that are artful additions to the gardens where they reside. Make one as a family project, then observe who moves in over time.

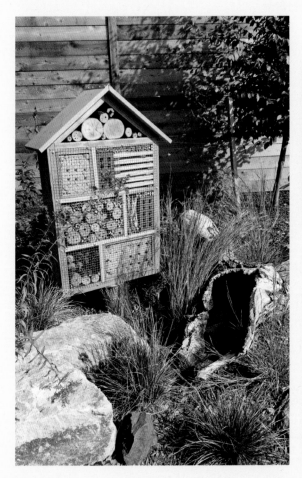

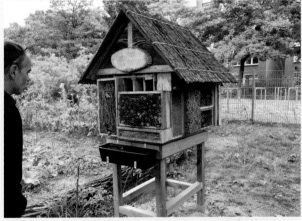

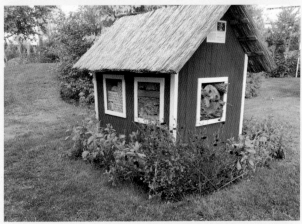

Making a home for native bees

There are more than 1300 species of native, cavity-dwelling bees in North America, and they are important pollinators. They don't produce honey, but they do pollinate at least 30 percent of our food crops and up to 90 percent of native plants. These bees may live near each other, but not in hives like honeybees (which have a queen and worker bees), so native bees are considered solitary bees. The males do not have stingers and the females only sting when trapped or squeezed; because they pose little risk of stinging, these valuable pollinators make good neighbors.

Each native mama bee builds her own nest and stocks it with special food for her babies. If you wish to attract these essential pollinators, placing your insect hotel in or near flower beds will ensure that mother bees have access to the pollen and nectar they need to feed their babies. Be sure you have native flowers and the flowers of fruit trees in bloom for the entire time bees are active: early March through late June in most places. Mason bees lay their eggs in hollow tubes and tunnels. Your insect hotel will provide an abundance of these nesting spots, so that bees are encouraged to live in and pollinate your garden.

If your hotel will have wooden nest blocks, be sure to use preservative-free wood. You can drill into logs and sticks or lumber blocks. Bees don't like the inside of their tunnels to be rough, so use a sharp bit, and drill with the grain, not across it. Drill tunnels between ³⁄₃₂ inch and ³⁄₈ inch in diameter. It is recommended that you stick to one diameter per block or per section—however, change up hole sizes and depths in other sections to attract a variety of bees and other insects that are active throughout the year.

To most effectively attract the bees you want, try to mimic the conditions that bees look for in nature. Tunnels that are less than ¼ inch in diameter should be 3 to 5 inches deep. Tunnels larger than ¼ inch should be 5 to 6 inches deep (if you can drill that far). Leave at least ¾ inch between each hole. Bees don't nest in tunnels that are open all the way through, so tunnels and tubes intended for bees in your insect hotel need to be closed at one end. Bees also like their houses to be dry. An overhanging roof helps keep rain out.

Bees prefer houses that are warm but not too hot. They like morning sun, so face your insect hotel south or southeast for the morning sun, but locate it in a spot that will get afternoon shade. Other insects prefer shadier, damper nesting spaces. A two-sided hotel will accommodate everyone. You may want to mount the insect hotel on a pole or tree 3 to 6 feet off the ground,

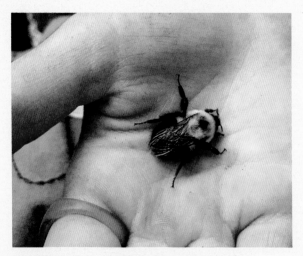

Native bees don't make honey, but are essential for pollination.

but it can also be set in a dry spot on the ground. Don't place your hotel near bird feeders. That can make it too inviting for birds to bother the bees.

Native bee nesting and reproduction

A mother bee will first head to the farthest back portion of the nesting tunnel. She will stock the space with special baby bee food, a blend of pollen and nectar, then lay one egg, and build a little wall to tuck that baby in safely. Different kinds of bees use different materials to build their walls, so you may see leaves, mud, or even a special kind of bee spit that dries into a hard surface. The eggs of female babies are laid back in the deepest part of the tunnel (more than 3 inches deep) and the eggs of male babies are laid in the front 3 inches of the tunnel. To be sure your hotel produces lots of baby bees of both genders, make sure the holes are as deep as possible.

The mother bee keeps laying eggs and building walls until she has filled the tunnel with 5 to 8 eggs. She then moves on to another tunnel and continues this until the season ends or she dies. Some tunnels may be only partially filled. Because of this, you may not be able to tell which tunnels have babies inside, even if you look very carefully down into the tunnel.

What is happening inside? After about a week, a larva hatches from an egg. The larva eats the food that mama left, and after another week, spins a cocoon. In the fall, the pupa emerges from that cocoon and, still in the nest, transforms into an adult bee. The adult hibernates in that same nest until spring, when the bees chew their way out of their little cell in the nest. Males, whom you'll recall are living in the front of the tube,

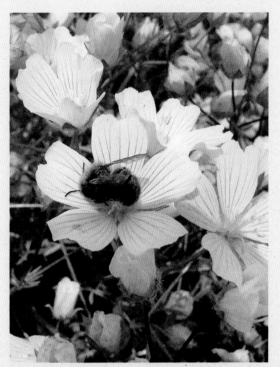

A female mason bee tends to her food-gathering and pollination duties.

emerge first and wait outside the door for the females to emerge. They mate, and the whole process begins again.

Some species of mother mason bees need mud to close off each egg chamber. If your soil is too sandy, the bees won't use it, and won't be able to occupy your hotel. So provide the amenities that bees need: a pile of damp to wet, clayey soil somewhere nearby.

Large numbers of bees nesting in a small space can attract unwanted guests such as parasites and fungi. Bees aren't good at recognizing a clean or dirty hotel, so it's your job to get rid of old nesting materials and replace them with fresh, new materials. Clean out your hotel every year or two to avoid infestations of parasites and the spread of other diseases. One of the advantages of a mixed insect hotel is that some of the other insects who may reside there will be good at exterminating the parasites that might attack bees. These bee allies include lacewings, ladybugs, beetles, and earwigs.

More information on creating wildlife-friendly spaces

Besides the tips offered in *Bringing Nature Home*, the National Wildlife Federation (NWF), the National Audubon Society, and the Cornell Lab of Ornithology also offer information for making your backyard attractive to wildlife and for helping kids learn about birds and other backyard creatures (see Resources section). One goal of these organizations is to replace diminishing habitat for wildlife by encouraging people to transform their home landscapes with native plants, so that they can become part of the habitat corridors that wildlife need.

The NWF offers a certification for backyards and schoolyards that are wildlife friendly. Their program asks that certified spaces provide all the habitat components that meet the needs of wildlife. These components include food (such as seeds, berries, suet, pollen, nuts), water (a birdbath, butterfly puddle, pond, or nearby stream), cover (shrubs, birdhouses, brush piles), and places for wildlife to raise their young (such as a dead tree, a nearby meadow, or a butterfly's host plant). They also ask that you employ sustainable practices in your site, such as reducing the amount of lawn. For more information, visit NWF.org.

Don't Let Fears Keep Kids Homebound

There are real dangers in the world, and real reasons to be afraid sometimes. Children encounter these and process them daily. By talking to children about their fears and by exposing them to new places and experiences, we help them to develop realistic understandings of the world.

Many of us worry about the dangers of nature. We can help children to confront fears they may have about nature or wildlife with knowledge. It is essential to be mindful of what we are modeling for children, because they learn more from watching what adults do than from listening to what adults say, especially if the two contradict. When it comes to nature, we should be modeling curiosity, understanding, and reasonable caution—not phobias or repulsion.

It is important to protect children from serious injury (which can be defined as an injury from which one cannot heal), to take reasonable precautions, and to be thoughtful and realistic about risk. This needs to be balanced with an acknowledgment of the value and benefits of risk—a few mosquito bites or a scraped knee is a reasonable trade-off for helping kids develop resilience and confidence outdoors.

Plants That Naturally Repel Biting Insects

Insect bites rank high on many people's list of fears. Stinging insects like bees, wasps, and mosquitoes, as well as ticks that can carry disease, create a great deal of concern. The following plants can help create a yard where bite-free zones can coexist with insect hotels, bee houses, and other insect habitat.

Catnip (*Nepeta cataria*)
Citronella grass (*Cymbopogon nardus* and *C. winterianus*)
Citronella-scented geranium (*Pelargonium citrosum*)
Lemon balm (*Melissa officinalis*)
Lemon eucalyptus (*Corymbia citriodora*)
Lemongrass (*Cymbopogon*)
Marigold (*Tagetes*)
Mosquito plant (*Pelargonium citronellum*)
Peppermint (*Mentha × piperita*)
Rosemary (*Rosmarinus officinalis*)

Avoiding Insect Bites and Critter Calamities

+ **Spread cedar mulch** in your play space. It is a natural insecticide, and it smells great.

+ **Get rid of standing water,** even small amounts. Be sure to cover the overflow pipe from your rain barrels with screening so mosquitoes can't get inside. Wherever there is unavoidable standing water, use mosquito dunks, a non-toxic (to fish, animals, and people) cake that prevents mosquito larvae from hatching. It is available at hardware stores and garden shops.

+ **Welcome the wildlife that feeds on insects.** They will do their job to help reduce the population of annoying bugs. Bat houses, toad houses, birdhouses, and insect hotels all help invite the predators needed to keep pests under control.

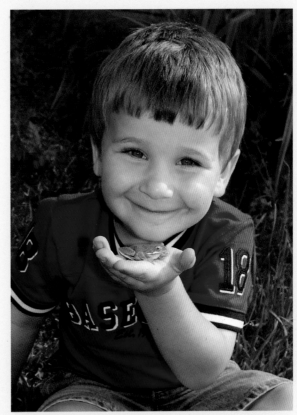

Caution is always important, but kids should learn that nature is a place of wonder and fun surprises.

+ **Watch for ticks.** Unfortunately, deer bring ticks and ticks can bring disease. If you can surround your site with tall fencing, you will protect your plants from hungry deer, and reduce the tick population as well. Besides providing fresh eggs, pet chickens love to dine on ticks, so keeping hens (or any ground-dwelling birds) will help control the population of ticks and other insects. If you're in a place with tall grass, where ticks like to hang out, take precautions. Wear long pants tucked into your socks or boots. Wear light colors so you can see ticks on your clothing. Go over your clothing with an adhesive lint roller periodically. It will grab ticks before they have a chance to grab you. Inspect children from head to toe as part of your daily routine after an outing where ticks might have been. Deer ticks are tiny; learn to identify them.

+ **Use insect repellent.** It can be made of natural materials like catmint, lemon eucalyptus, peppermint oil, citronella, and other strong-smelling herbs, so that it is not toxic on children's skin but helps keep bugs away. You can also buy clothing impregnated with insect repellant. If you feel you must use repellent containing Deet, only spray it on clothing. Research tells us that catmint and lemon eucalyptus are both *more effective than Deet* at repelling disease-carrying insects. Use insect repellent with caution, however, whether it is natural or not. Be scrupulous in avoiding contact with eyes. Repellent, especially the natural types, may need to be reapplied if you're out for a long time.

+ **Take necessary allergy precautions** for any child who could have a serious reaction, but under normal circumstances, try not to fuel fright. Children need to learn that some insects sting (and why), but the use of repellent and having bite-free zones of repellent plants should allow kids to feel relatively safe in their outdoor play. One colleague of mine transformed the outdoor space at their childcare center from an equipment-based space to a natural play space. As required by local regulations, staff workers were diligent about documenting accidents and injuries. A surprising discovery was that although the newly planted native plants were attracting a range of pollinators and beneficial insects, the accident and injury reports showed that there were *fewer* bee stings after the natural play space went in. The theory was that the bees were too busy in their welcoming habitat to spend time stinging humans. I'm not sure if that's scientifically accurate, but it is evidence to calm those for whom the sight of a bee is frightening.

+ **Teach about snakes.** It's important to learn the venomous snakes that might live in your region and to make sure children know how to recognize them and stay away. But if you yourself carry a primal but irrational fear, don't transfer it to children exhibiting a natural and healthy interest in snakes and other wild creatures. Teach kids to observe and to touch gently. Knowledge helps build respect and empathy for those who share their homes with us. Visit your local nature center, where staff may be willing to take a gentle and harmless snake out and allow children to stroke and possibly hold it. First-hand experience leads to understanding—the best antidote to fear.

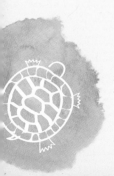

PLANTS for A BUTTERFLY-FRIENDLY YARD

ALMOST EVERY PLANT ON THIS LIST is a native that evolved right along with the butterflies whose babies depend on it for food. Watch out for non-natives and especially invasive plants such as butterfly bush (*Buddlea*), which attracts clouds of butterflies for its "junk food" nectar. Your butterflies deserve the best. Plant natives!

COMMON NAME	BOTANICAL NAME	LEAVES FEED THESE CATERPILLARS	NECTAR FEEDS THESE ADULT BUTTERFLIES	DESCRIPTION
Aster	*Aster* species	Pearl crescent		Perennial flower that blooms in summer and early fall.
Black locust	*Robinia pseudoacacia*	Silver-spotted skippers		Tall overstory tree.
Blueberries	*Vaccinium* species	Brown and hoary elfins		Shrub for sun or shade, with bright red fall color (and yummy berries).
Common boneset	*Eupatorium perfoliatum*		Multiple	Perennial flower that grows in beautiful groves.
Dutchman's pipevine	*Aristolochia macrophylla*	Pipevine swallowtail		Vine that blooms purple in late spring and early summer.
Eastern pine	*Pinus strobus*	Elfin		Conifer tree with long, soft needles.
Eastern red cedar	*Juniperus virginiana*	Olive juniper hairstreak		Evergreen tree.
Goldenrod	*Solidago* varieties		Multiple	Perennial with yellow flowers in fall.
Ironweed	*Vernonia noveboracensis*		Multiple	Purple flowering perennial in late summer and fall.
Milkweed	*Asclepias* species	Monarch	Multiple	Perennial that flowers in early summer. Likes medium to moist soil.
Mountain mint	*Pycnanthemum muticum*		Multiple	Herbaceous perennial that grows in part sun with minty scented leaves.

COMMON NAME	BOTANICAL NAME	LEAVES FEED THESE CATERPILLARS	NECTAR FEEDS THESE ADULT BUTTERFLIES	DESCRIPTION
Oak	*Quercus* species	Hairstreak and others		Large shade tree that produces acorns.
Pawpaw	*Asimina triloba*	Zebra swallowtail		Small tree that grows in sun or shade and produces delicious fruit.
Pearly everlasting	*Anaphalis margaritacea*	American lady		White-flowering perennial with silvery foliage. Likes dry sunny spots.
Prairie gay feather	*Liatris spicata*		Multiple	Perennial with spikey purple flowers in summer.
Pussy toes	*Antennaria parlinii*	American painted lady	Multiple	Fuzzy silvery leaves make a good ground cover. The pink or white flowers look like tiny cat feet.
Sassafras	*Sassafras albidum*	Swallowtail		Small tree with 3 different shaped leaf types on every plant, and beautiful yellow fall color.
Spicebush	*Lindera benzoin*	Spicebush swallowtail		Shrub that grows in shady spots. Yellow fall color.
Tulip poplar	*Liriodendron tulipifera*	Eastern tiger swallowtail		Very tall overstory tree for shade.
Violet	*Viola* species	Fritillary		Creeping ground cover in shade.
Wild carrot* and other members of the family Umbelliferae such as fennel, dill, parsley	*Daucus carota*	Black swallowtail		Naturalized from a European herb brought by settlers. A wild meadow plant.

*Indicates non-native. All other plants listed are North American natives.

Interacting with animals

Caring for animals, whether wildlife or pets, is enriching for children because it invites them to pay attention and observe. It teaches them to consider and respect others. There is tremendous value in having a living creature to love. The comfort of cuddling with a furry pet lowers blood pressure and reduces stress. There are wonderful programs that bring therapy dogs to children in schools, libraries, and parks so they can practice reading to a nonjudgmental audience. (I'm writing this book with my sweet, purring cat snuggled by my side.)

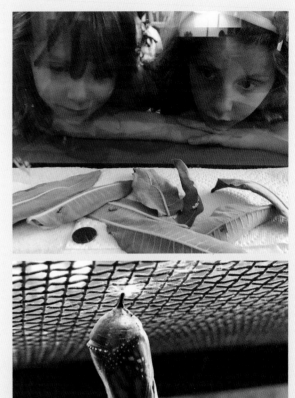

Hatching butterflies from caterpillars responsibly at home can help give endangered species like monarchs a head start against predators. A mesh container allows good air circulation. Be sure you have a plentiful supply of the kind of leaves your caterpillars like so you can serve fresh ones at least once a day. Clip off a stem and set it in a bottle of water to help keep leaves fresh longer. If kids are lucky, they'll get to witness a butterfly emerging from its cocoon.

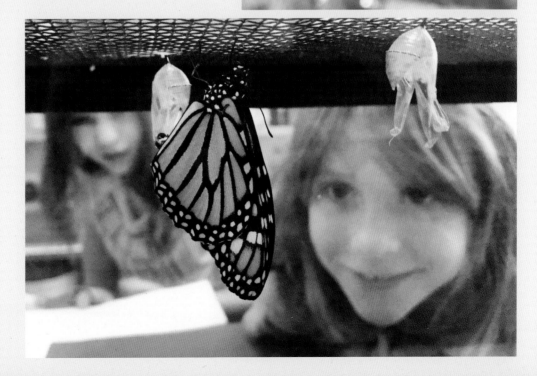

Everybody, people and pets included, needs some time outside in the fresh air and sunshine. In order to enjoy the outdoors with pets, there may need to be special places for them. Consider a fenced area to be safely outside with the family dog or cat, or a low pen that is big enough for a child or two to sit with their pet bunny or guinea pig, with grass for the furry friend to nibble. If you live in a place that permits it, think about keeping goats or chickens.

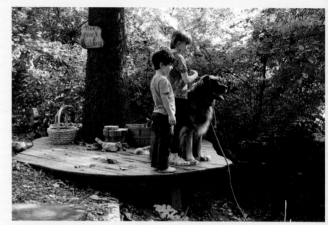

Kids and dogs growing up outdoors together helps keep everyone active.

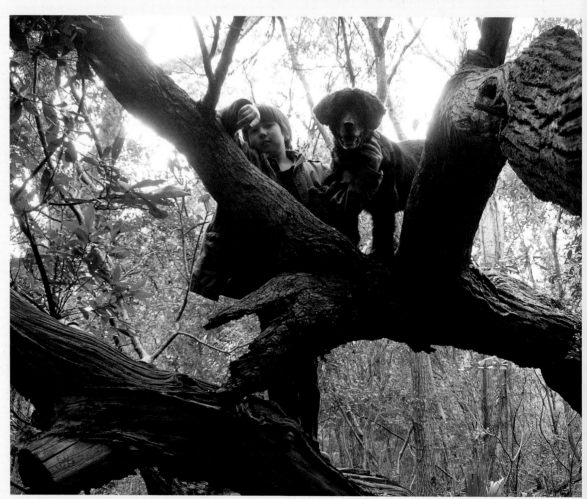

A loyal dog will accompany his favorite child on any adventure.

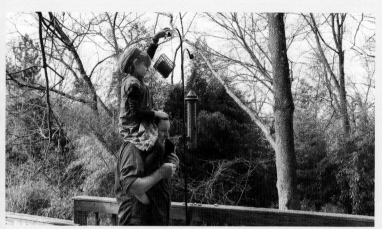

Think about views out the window into nature as well. A bird feeder can entertain even when the weather doesn't cooperate.

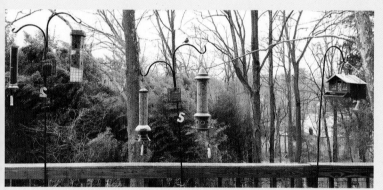

An assortment of bird feeders and food can become an experiment to compare which the birds prefer. (The numbers help make it easy to identify each feeder, in observations and in conversations.)

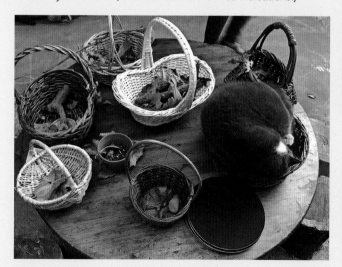

Kitty naps in a basket of nature discoveries.

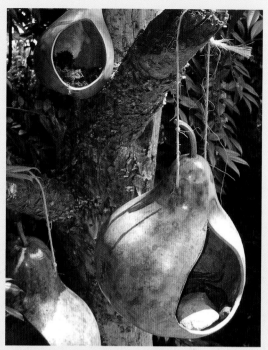

Grow birdhouse gourds in your garden, then harvest, let them dry out, cut openings, and hang them in the spring for nesting birds.

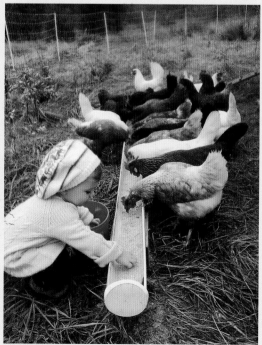

Even the littlest member of the family can help care for a flock of backyard chickens.

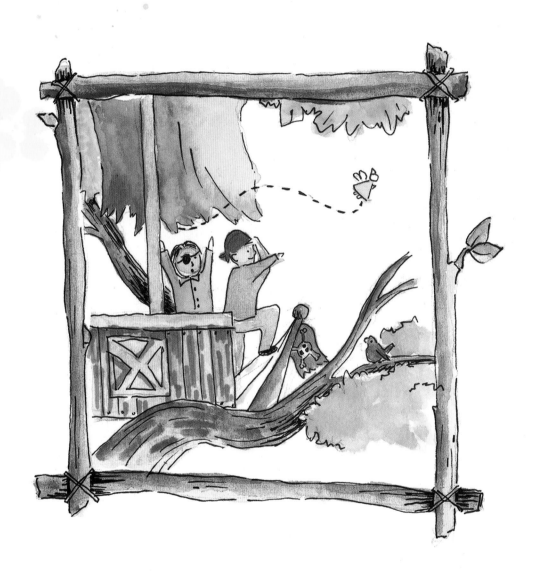

Inspiring Imagination

"Talking to trees and hiding in trees precedes saving trees."

—from *Childhood and Nature: Design Principles for Educators*, by David Sobel

Pretend play is the stuff of childhood, as well as an important foundation for healthy adulthood. Slipping into the role of doctor or dragon opens a magical doorway to important learning. Imagining oneself with knowledge, competence, and power beyond one's 4-year-old self leads a child to test what it feels like to be in charge, maybe to care for others, or to have control—and that helps develop confidence in one's abilities.

The free and unstructured outdoors is uniquely well suited to provide the sort of open-ended, pretend-play settings where imagination blossoms. Being together with friends, sheltered from weather, protected from danger, empowered to defeat the forces of evil are the themes of many dramatic play scenarios through which children explore what it means to be safe and have a home. Having control over these spaces, and the option to arrange and rearrange gives children a sense of ownership, of territory, and of their own power to create spaces that are comfortable and pleasing. Role playing with others allows kids to try on, practice, and master valuable social skills like conversation, negotiation, empathy, and cooperation.

By helping our children create outdoor settings for imaginary play, we give them tools to deeply explore fundamental issues of life, family, work, and community. Abundant time, inviting spaces, and peers to play with are the essential ingredients for imaginations to grow. Providing playful opportunities for our children to learn how to navigate social interactions, establish personal boundaries, and develop their own emotional intelligence is one of the most valuable gifts we can give our children.

MAGICAL HIDEAWAYS

If you've ever had the experience of returning as an adult to a place where you spent time as a child, you know that scale matters. As you grew, the cavernous place you remember from childhood didn't shrink, but it seemed like it did. This memory can help us understand how even standard-sized spaces can seem very big to a small child. It also helps us to understand the value of low-ceilinged, child-sized spaces, which feel especially inviting to kids.

Our ancestors evolved in green places and found safety from predators and protection from the elements in natural shelters. Children are drawn to spaces where they can be enclosed for similar reasons. There is a deep, biologically based sense of protection and security that comes from being enclosed, enveloped, and hidden.

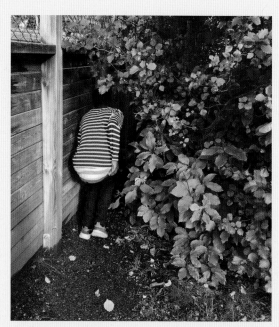

This secret spot is so small and hidden, an adult might not notice it. To a child like this one, however, it is an important haven.

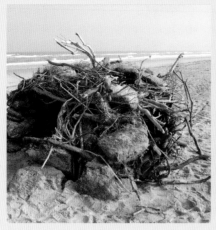

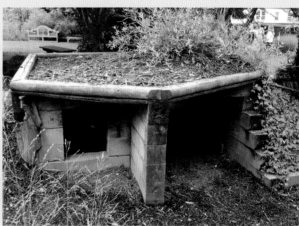

From a driftwood hut on the beach to a partially underground shelter, a stick house in the forest to a wattle-and-earth dome, children everywhere crave dens and hiding places.

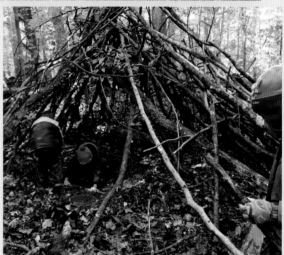

The stage for imaginary play can be ephemeral: a cozy igloo in the winter or autumn leaves raked to define rooms in a house. Sticks and other loose natural pieces can be the raw materials to create a nest for a family of pretend eagles, a teepee of Native Americans, the lean-to of a pioneer family, or a rocket bringing explorers to new frontiers.

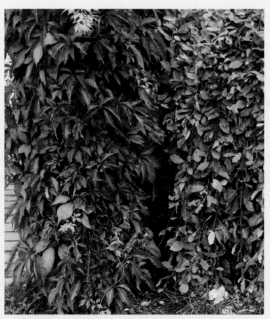

A hiding place in the leaves. See that sweet face peeking out?

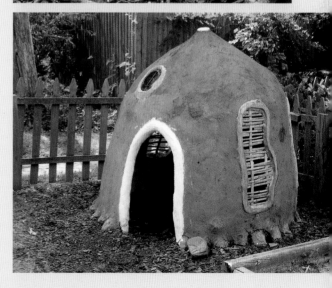

The experience of playing among the leafy branches of a grove of lilacs, beneath a weeping willow, or under a low-branching magnolia creates powerful memories that you may have from your own childhood. The branches of trees create a sense of enclosure and safety, perhaps reminiscent of what our prehistoric ancestors felt when they found safe harbor among trees on the savannah. These outdoor rooms ignite imaginations and are the settings for stories and worlds to be created.

Weeping trees, living willow structures, clusters of grasses or shrubs, arbors, bowers, and open-framed playhouses planted with vines—all provide the magic of being surrounded by an enclosure made of greenery. There are times when we all need to be alone, and for some that need is strong. Time away from others allows us to relax, retreat, and restore ourselves. It is important to offer inviting natural spaces that provide children some respite from the noise and negotiations that come with city living or group care. We can create these small, enclosed niches with a seat or perch just big enough for one. If you have more than one child in your play space, having more than one private space is a good idea. Furnishings like work surfaces, seating, and props can add richness to stories and their play. Add child-sized log tables, chairs, benches, dishes, and tools made of natural materials. Don't forget dress-up clothes and costumes.

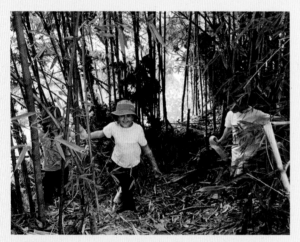

This clearing in a bamboo grove is a favorite destination for adventurous play in all seasons.

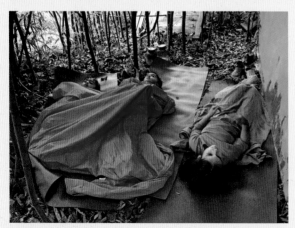

When mats and blankets are added, it is perfect for a cozy rest.

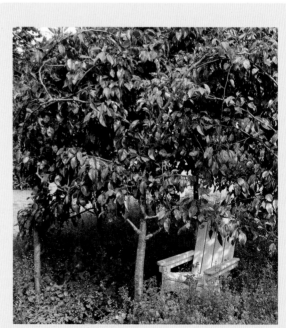

A shaded seat just big enough for one offers the opportunity for some time alone.

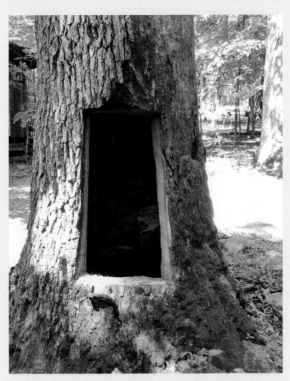

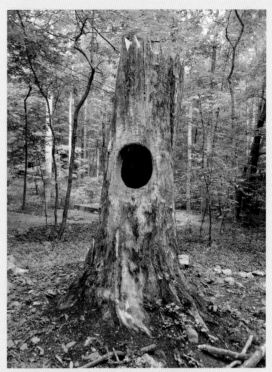

Hollow trees are such perfect invitations to imagine. Here a hollow stump about 8 feet tall was left when the rest of the tree was removed. It was then enhanced by some creative work with a saw. A square entry door is one side.

The other side of the hollow stump has a peeking-out window. Whimsical spikes were carved into the top.

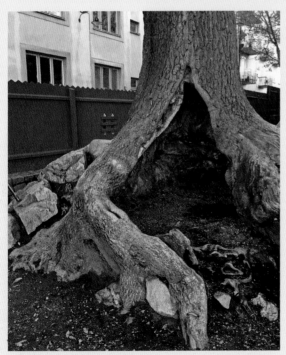

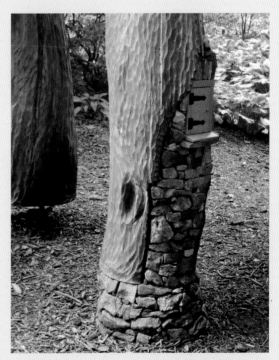

Hollow trunks invite stories of who might live there. A fairy? A fox?

One leg of this hollow tree has been embellished with stonework and a tiny door.

Lots of tree species have weeping varieties. Under these canopies are perfect places to get that cozy sense of being surrounded by greenery. Hiding out in a grove of shrubs is another way to create that feeling. Some shrubs, especially natives, grow in colonies, which means their spreading roots send up shoots and become new nearby shrubs. All the plants in the accompanying list will provide great green enclosures for play.

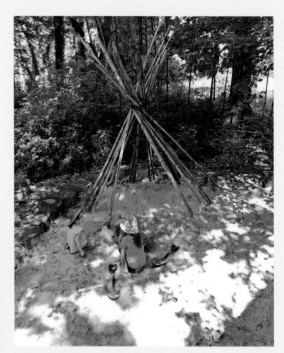

Pole huts provide just the right amount of enclosure—with a view.

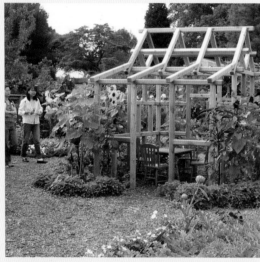

This playhouse structure is open enough for views in and out, while still defining an interior space.

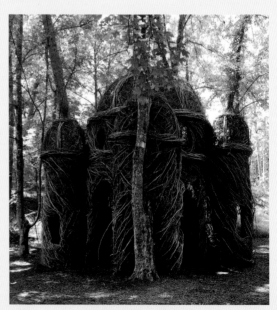

A bewitching castle made of saplings surprises travelers on the riverwalk in Hillsborough, North Carolina. It is the work of artists Patrick Dougherty and Elsa Hoffman, along with over one hundred volunteers.

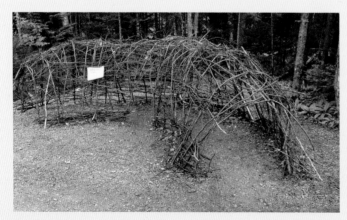

Raw materials are everywhere. Encountering this twigwork sculpture in the forest lets us believe that the wood nymphs have been building.

Weeping Trees and Sculptable Shrubs for Hiding Places

Lilac* (*Syringa* species) Lilacs, once established, colonize out from the center, leaving open spaces in the middle that are perfect for play. The fragrance of lilac blooms in the spring will stay with you throughout your life and carry grown-up you right back to childhood whenever you encounter it.

Summersweet (*Clethra alnifolia*) Spreading by underground shoots, summersweet forms groves that can be hollowed out in the center to create a room for play. Summersweet produces fragrant pink or white flowers in midsummer and has yellow fall color.

Sweetshrub (*Calycanthus floridus*) Sweetshrub colonizes in moist soil and leaves open spaces that are perfect for hiding out and pretending. The pickable early summer flowers look like they are carved from wood and produce a unique sour apple scent that kids love.

Sweetspire (*Itea virginica*) Corkscrew-shaped white flower bundles appear in spring and the leaves turn a spectacular bright red in fall. Sweetspire spreads and multiplies, so it's the perfect shrub in which to create a leafy play niche. For a head start, plant it in groups.

Weeping cherry* (*Prunus* species) Can grow to be very large. In spring, huddling under the cascade of pink blossoms is like being transported to another world.

Weeping pussy willow* (*Salix caprea* 'Pendula') Soft, furry catkins appear in spring, so just being near this sweet, diminutive tree is soothing.

Weeping willow* (*Salix babylonica*) The largest of the weeping trees. Being underneath this spectacular canopy is a powerful experience. Weeping willow loves a wet spot.

Weeping beech* (*Fagus sylvatica* 'Pendula') Cascading branches of weeping beech can enclose a room-sized space below.

Weeping katsura* (*Cercidiphyllum japonicum* 'Pendulum') At its most spectacular in autumn, weeping katsura leaves turn vibrant gold and release a fragrance that will remind you of brown sugar and maple syrup.

Weeping redbud (*Cercis canadensis* 'Covey' or 'Lavender Twist') A small to medium-sized native tree with a waterfall of (edible!) purple blooms in spring.

*Indicates non-native. All other plants listed are North American natives.

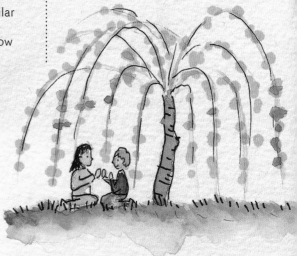

A LIVING WILLOW TUNNEL

Living willow whips can be planted around the footprint of a space you want to enclose. As they grow, which they do very quickly, whips can be woven together to create tunnels, fedges (a living fence-hedge), and bowers.

   This is a project for early spring, when the willow you'll need is in abundant supply and has the best potential to take root easily. What follows are basic instructions. There are volumes written about this topic, especially from the United Kingdom, where it is a highly evolved form of landscape art. Start small, dream big, and see where this nature sculpting takes you.

   Almost any type of willow will work. I've cut branches from willows growing wild along a nearby creek. Some nice North American native varieties include American pussy willow (*Salix discolor*), bluestem willow (*Salix irrorata*, native to southeastern U.S.), eastern black willow (*Salix nigra*), and woolly headed willow (*Salix eriocephala*).

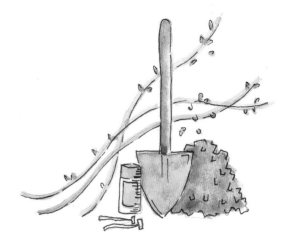

WHAT YOU'LL NEED

* landscape-marking spray paint
* willow whips (long, slender cuttings of willow branches) in varying diameters. As for length, 8 to 10 feet is ideal, but you can work with any length because they will grow! You will need about 3 whips per foot of perimeter.
* shovel
* cable or twist ties
* mulch

1 Start this project in early spring, so the willow starts will have the summer to get established and can be tied and completed by late summer or early autumn.

2 Choose a level spot.

3 Use spray paint to mark the outline of the structure you want to build (tunnel, dome, bower, fedge).

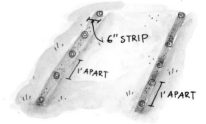

4 Set your heaviest willow whips 1 foot into the ground and spaced 1 foot apart around the perimeter of your structure. Don't forget to leave an opening for the door. The whips may be small to start. In that case you can let them grow for a while and continue with the following steps when the whips are at least 2 to 3 feet long.

6" STRIP

1' APART

1' APART

5 Go around the perimeter, adding secondary, smaller whips tilted at 45 degrees. Then add one more layer of whips, angled at 45 degrees in the opposite direction. Weave the diagonal willow whips over and under and across the structure. Secure with cable ties.

6 In order to grow roots, the whips need to be kept constantly moist. You can water diligently or install drip irrigation around the perimeter.

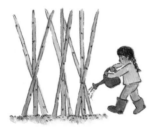

7 Mulch 6 inches around each of the willow whips to keep weeds away from the structure. You can use straw, wood chips, or leaves.

8 When the whips get tall enough, fasten them together to form a ceiling and create an enclosed space below.

9 Keep paying attention to the willow whips as they grow and send out new branches. Weave these new branches into the structure before they get too big and stiff.

10 Trim off stray branches to keep the shape of your structure.

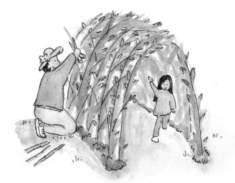

11 Plant the trimmed pieces to fill in any gaps where a whip may have died.

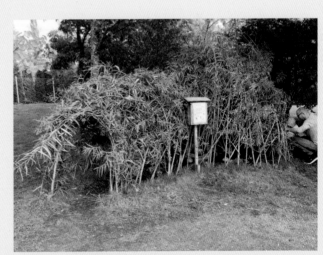

A living willow tunnel leading to a round room at the Botanical Garden of Uppsala in Sweden.

BASIC WOODEN POST HUT

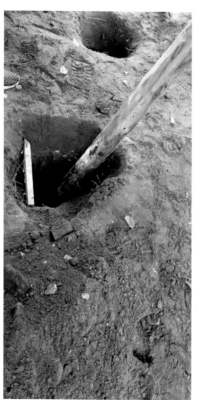 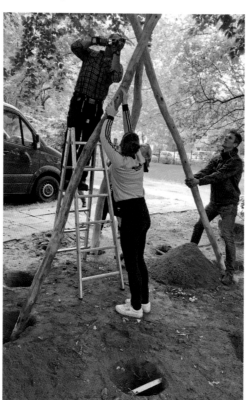 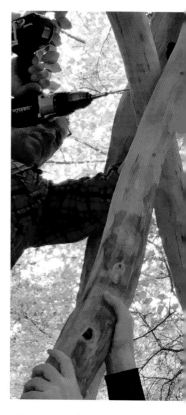

1   Start with 6 to 8 stripped locust posts. Dig evenly spaced holes in a circle.

2   Set posts in holes.

3   Anchor the top with screws.

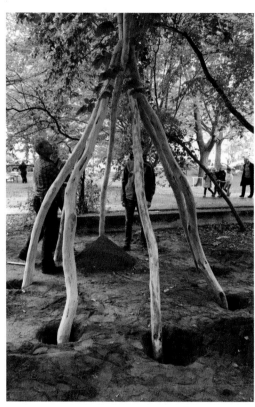

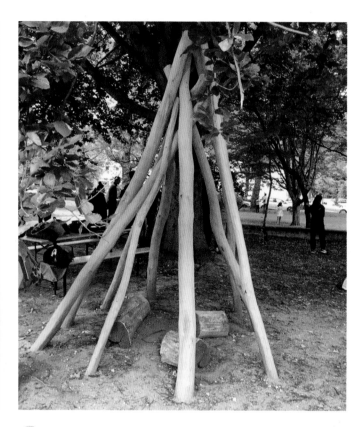

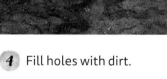 **4** Fill holes with dirt.

5 Ready for play! Skeleton structures suggest enclosure on their own, and can be embellished with randomly wound yarn, ribbons, vines, fabric, or blankets to increase the sense of enclosure.

CHILD-SIZED ELEMENTS

It is important to provide places to play that are scaled to the way a child sees the world. A playhouse can be a more long-term addition to your play space that is perfectly sized for imaginary play. Consider the dimensions of windows, chairs, and tables, and the height of doorknobs and countertops. When a play setting is scaled to child proportions, it fosters the ability to imagine oneself a grown-up, doing important jobs. Hinged doors and shutters that children can open and close (designed carefully to avoid pinch points) appeal to young children's drive to experiment with mechanical devices and provide a satisfying way to define one's territory.

If there is more than one child using the play space, consider ways to provide for "village play." This could mean having two playhouses—which increases the play value by more than double. Having a village adds new dimensions and roles to games, encourages language and social interactions, and increases the amount of movement and physical activity that happens.

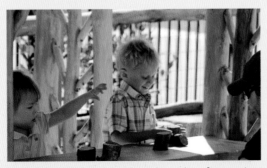

Realistic child-sized props can enhance play, as in this playhouse with Dutch doors and dishes for a tea party.

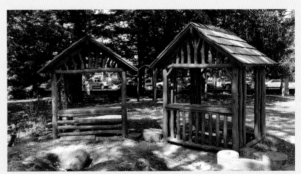

Two playhouses can foster village play among small or large groups of kids. Open twigwork lets children feel enclosed but gives adults a view in.

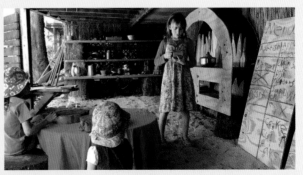

Pass-through windows and a wide work surface are just the thing for "cooking," conversation, and cooperation.

An oven cutout complete with flames, a guest table and tablecloth, and a child-made menu board let these friends explore a restaurant theme.

Living roofs soften man-made structures in a natural play space, connect them to nature, and provide some habitat and green space in a surprising place. Children can be involved in choosing and planting the plants. The low roof of a playhouse makes the plants especially visible.

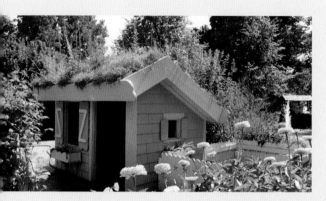

This playhouse with a living, thriving roof makes nature part of the fun.

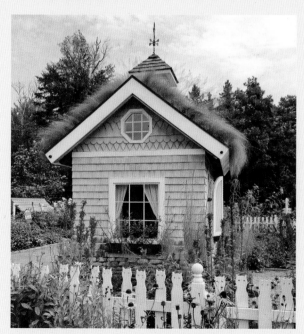

Another advantage of living-roof playhouses is that, when insulated, they can be a cool hideout on hot summer days.

Ten Plants for a Colorful, Kid-Friendly Living Roof

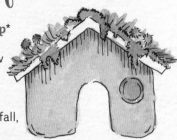

'Angelina' stonecrop* (*Sedum rupestre* 'Angelina') Rainbow foliage transforms from lime green in spring to yellow in summer, orange in fall, and red in winter.

'Blue spruce' stonecrop* (*Sedum reflexum* 'Blue Spruce') Like a tiny tree, this plant has beautiful silver-blue foliage all year, and bright yellow flowers on tall spikes in midsummer.

Chives* (*Allium schoenoprasum*) Purple pom-pom flowers appear in late spring. The plant is onion scented.

Crocus* (*Crocus* species) Purple, blue, yellow, and white flowers pop up in early spring.

'Golden carpet' stonecrop* (*Phedimus takesimensis* 'Golden Carpet') A nearly evergreen plant that attracts butterflies with an early-spring carpet of yellow flowers.

Grape hyacinth* (*Muscari armeniacum*) Fragrant blue or white flowers bloom in midspring.

Hens and chickens* (*Sempervivum*) This popular plant forms spikey textured colonies of tiny and giant rosettes.

Ice plant* (*Delosperma cooperi*) A succulent with bright magenta flowers that bloom all summer on low foliage.

White stonecrop* (*Sedum album*) Striking leaves turn bright red in fall, winter, and spring. Tiny white flowers bloom in summer.

Fame flower (*Talinum calycinum*) Expect tall, wiry stems topped by pink flowers that open each afternoon from early summer to first frost. Easy to see from the ground.

*Indicates non-native. All other plants listed are North American natives.

PRETEND ANIMALS AND VEHICLES

Large natural elements like a gnarly log or a sculptural boulder are valuable for their open-endedness and flexibility. They can become whatever a child imagines them to be in the moment. Adding an element to the space that clearly represents an animal or a vehicle is less open-ended, but the details it provides can spur complexity in a child's play. When artfully constructed of natural materials, these features can fit into the space aesthetically and infuse whimsy and personality.

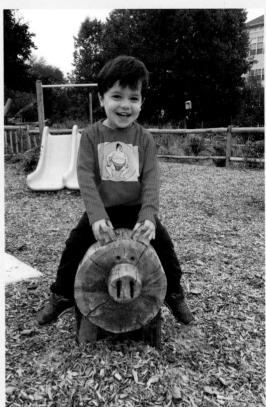

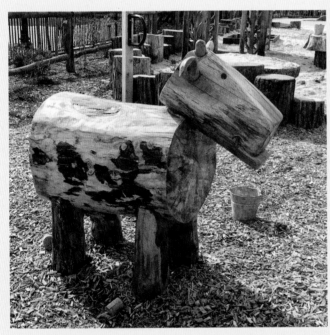

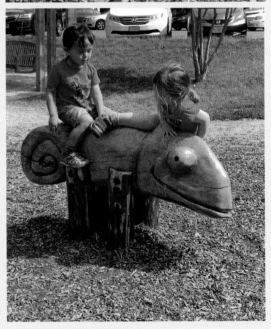

Climbable carved wooden animals inspire a wide range of play, from climbing and riding to conversation. Gathering hay for the sheep or pony, checking on the animals, and making sure they are warm and comfortable are all ways children practice caregiving.

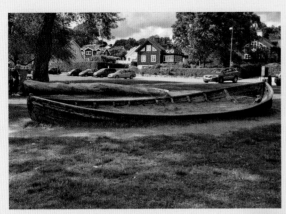

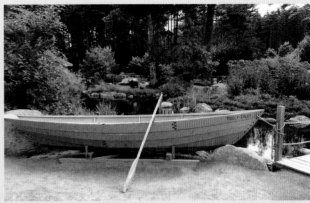

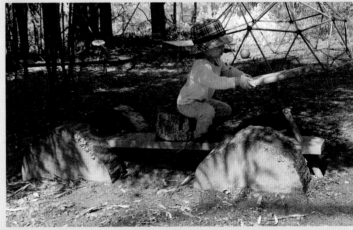

Confidence and empowerment come with access to stuff from the world of grown-ups, such as life-sized vehicles for pretending. Sailing a boat or driving a tractor are ways for children to experience a sense of control. Having a vehicle in the play space allows children to take imaginary journeys.

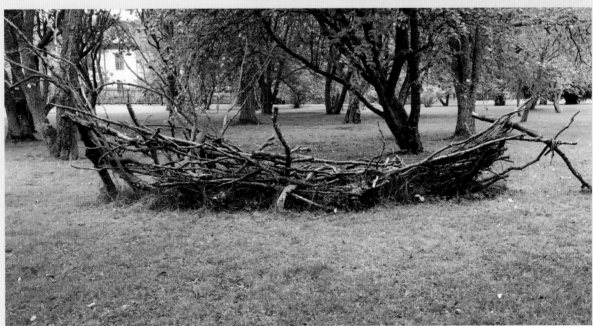

PERFORMANCE STAGES

The opportunity to perform before an audience, even an imaginary one, brings out the performer in a child. A simple outdoor platform, even at ground level or just one step up, provides a defined space for young actors, singers, musicians, magicians, and dancers. Costumes, props, and musical instruments enhance the performances. Imagination is used in different ways when children are improvising and playacting. Developing confidence in front of an audience is an important level of social-emotional learning.

Seating around the stage can provide a place for an audience, or for storytellers, actors, or musicians to perform. Consider adding a backdrop of simple plywood covered in chalkboard paint so children can easily draw scenes and change them. Seating can be sloped up a hillside, as with a natural amphitheater. A stage and seating under the shade of a big tree makes outdoor performances more comfortable in summer.

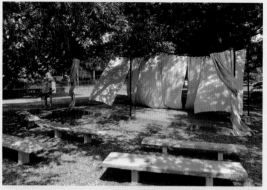

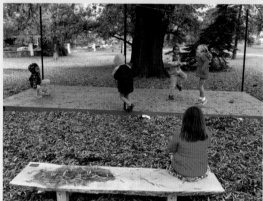

This is a place for singing, dancing, acting, and performances of both the official and improvised type, especially during summer. Removable curtains allow for simple changes in scenes and performers (top). But even in months when temperatures dip and curtains are gone, the shows go on (above).

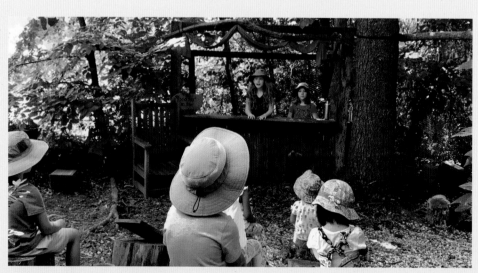

A puppet stage and stumps for audience seating give children a chance to be stars.

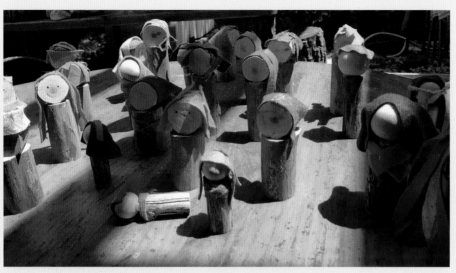
The "people" who populate tiny scenes can be figures made from natural materials.

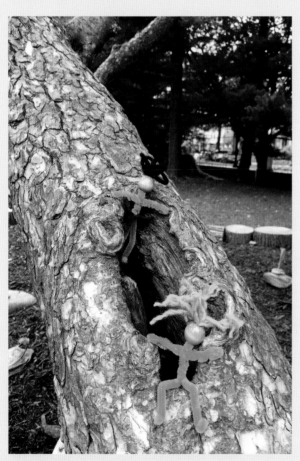
Yarn, pipe cleaners, and a leaning tree create an adventure for tiny climbers.

PLAY IN MINIATURE

Allowing children to create a tiny world provides a chance to imagine, tell stories, sort out complexity, and test theories of how people and the world work. It can help kids resolve challenging issues they may be facing. It can also be just plain fun!

There are all sorts of ways to support this kind of play outside. You and your child can set up a place for miniature world pretending. Bring some figures from indoor play (people from a dollhouse, Legos or Playmobil toys, or miniature animals) and play with them in the sandpit, the grass, or a planting bed. If you have flower pots on your deck or balcony, it's not hard to transform them with a few pebbles, sticks, and figures. Or create a special flower-pot fairy garden. It can be as elaborate as desired, with paths, buildings, even furniture. A hot glue gun makes it incredibly easy to build all sorts of play props with sticks and acorn shells, bits of moss, and other items from nature. A cardboard box or tray can be used to hold a changeable diorama.

Your miniature world can be a special corner of the play space, defined by a log or boulder edge, and planted with some of the fairy garden plants in the accompanying list, stocked with natural and store-bought loose parts from the toybox indoors.

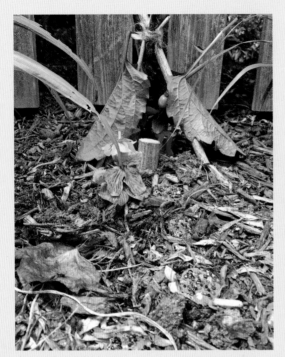

Beaded stepping stones lead to this leafy home.

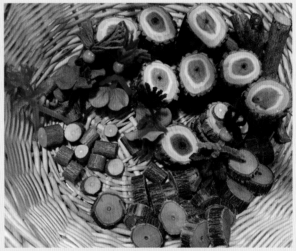

Tiny tree cookies make for a cozy setting. Some of the family members wear silk flower skirts.

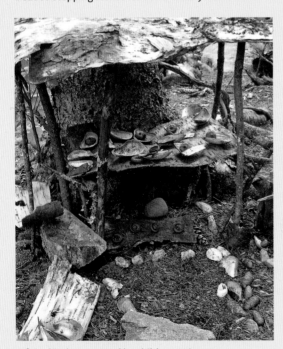

A fairy kitchen created by children, using natural materials.

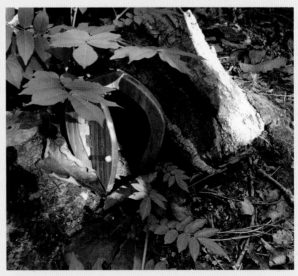

A door in a hollow tree sparks ideas about whose home this might be.

Plants for a Fairy or Giant Garden

Plants that have leaves or flowers at one extreme or the other in the size range are great for setting the scene and supporting imaginary play at different scales. Tiny plants carpeting the ground, shaded by an arching fern, are just right to enhance a garden for the smallest of fairies. At the other end of the spectrum, sometimes children like to imagine how it would feel to be a very small animal or imaginary creature. This helps them explore issues of power over the less powerful and to develop a sense of empathy. Trees and plants with giant leaves or flowers on very tall stalks help shift the scale of the world so it's easy to pretend to be a little mouse or a tiny fairy.

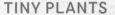

TINY PLANTS

Creeping Jenny* (*Lysimachia nummularia*) Bright yellow-green leaves are eye-catching, but watch this plant—it can be aggressive in some regions.

Dwarf crested iris (*Iris cristata*) A fairy garden favorite, growing only 3 to 6 inches tall.

Dwarf lady fern (*Athyrium filix-femina* 'Minutissimum') Lush 12-inch fern is perfect in part sun to full shade, tucked between rocks in a fairy garden.

Dwarf mondo grass* (*Ophiopogon japonicus* 'Nanus') A miniature version of the common ground cover, this one is only 2 to 3 inches tall.

Elfin thyme* (*Thymus serpyllum*) Teeny leaves are the hallmark of this low-growing, fragrant thyme.

Partridge berry (*Mitchella repens*) Mat-forming evergreen perennial that seldom gets more than 2 inches tall.

Pennsylvania sedge (*Carex pensylvanica*) Soft, arching, grasslike plant that makes a great no-mow lawn substitute in shade.

GIANT PLANTS

Bigleaf magnolia (*Magnolia macrophylla*), **umbrella magnolia** (*Magnolia tripetala*) Both of these trees have giant (1- to 2-foot-long) tropical leaves.

Ironweed (*Vernonia noveboracensis*) Features magenta-purple flowers on stalks 6 feet tall or higher.

Joe Pye weed (*Eutrochium purpueum*) Pinkish purple flowers bloom on stalks 6 feet tall or higher.

Ostrich fern (*Matteuccia struthiopteris*) Large, arching fronds grow 4 to 6 feet tall.

Pawpaw (*Asimina triloba*) Leaves can grow to 1 foot, helping make pawpaw seem like a plant from the jungle.

Swamp rosemallow (*Hibiscus moscheutos*) Look for dinner-plate-sized flowers 12 to 18 inches in diameter in shades of red, white, and pink.

Turkey foot grass (*Andropogon gerardii*) In a sunny spot, this grass can be 8 feet tall; foliage changes color with the seasons.

*Indicates non-native. All other plants listed are North American natives.

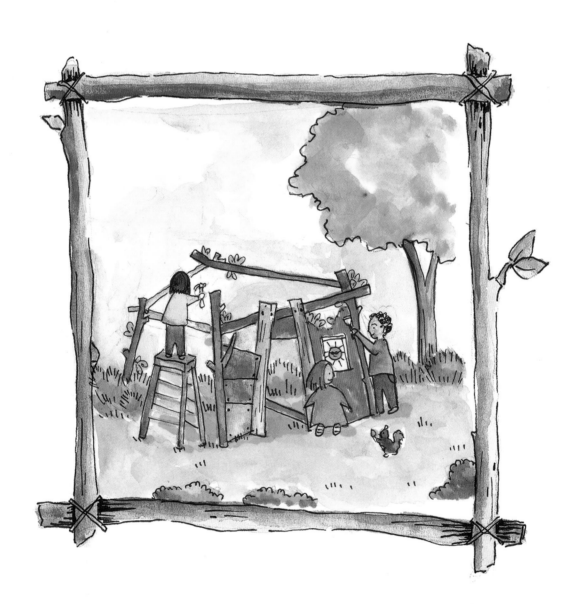

BUILDING CONFIDENCE

"Children need to have abundant time outdoors . . .
to construct a place and then play in it, or to get
into problem-solving on a big scale."

—from *Playing and Learning Outdoors*, by Jan White

C onfidence comes when children feel empowered, and there are few experiences more empowering than having the opportunity to build and create. These opportunities support many of the developmental tasks of childhood: being industrious and imaginative, building large and small muscles, learning language and cooperation—and acquiring the essential qualities of confidence and self-esteem.

To help children accomplish these milestones, supply elements in your outdoor space that kids can move around and use for constructing. Such materials are sometimes called "loose parts." And remember, in the out-of-doors, it's okay for the process of building things to be large scale and messy.

THE THEORY OF LOOSE PARTS

Raw materials offer tremendous play value and allow children to satisfy primitive drives—to build shelters and enclosures; to stack, balance, rearrange, and move things; to experiment, discover, and figure things out; and to lift, push, pull, drag, and carry. Loose parts can support a whole range of activities, from large-scale engineering, creating, and building to intricate, imaginative fine motor play.

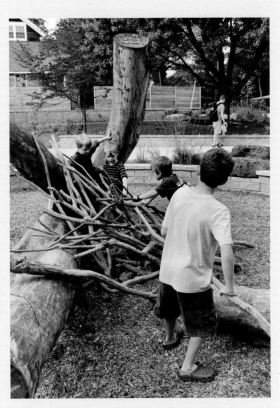

A group of ambitious children of all ages worked together to move a collection of sticks and then arrange them on this fallen tree. The project involved lots of lifting and climbing and heavy work to accomplish their goal.

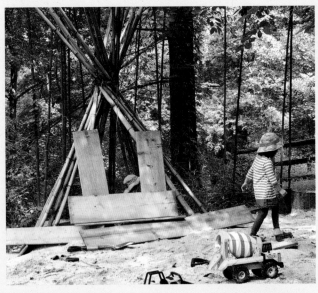

An open shelter can be embellished with a selection of materials to make it more enclosed. Here, boards have been carefully arranged by children to define their den.

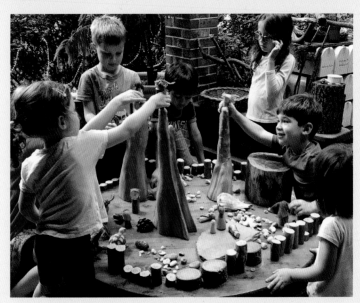

A play table stocked with natural materials (tiny tree cookies, stones, shells, and unique cypress knees) inspires intricate arranging and building.

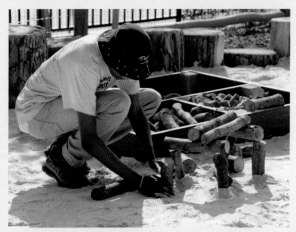

Loose parts engage kids of all ages.

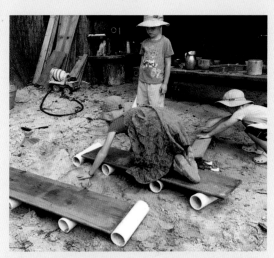

Lengths of PVC pipe and boards are transformed into a simple machine: a rolling board that can propel one across sand.

The theory of loose parts, put forth in a *Landscape Architecture* article titled "How NOT to Cheat Children: The Theory of Loose Parts" by Simon Nicholson in 1971, says that "in any environment, both the degree of inventiveness and creativity and the possibility of discovery are directly proportional to the *number and kind* of variables in the space." Nicholson was highly creative—a sculptor, an architect, and an advocate for children's right to agency and creativity. This theory of loose parts has influenced many schools of educational thought as well as designers around the world. The practical application of his theory is to have an abundance of things that children can move, arrange, and control in outdoor play spaces.

Loose parts allow children to satisfy their need to collect and gather, whether it be shells, acorns, pebbles and rocks, flowers, sticks, seed pods, or wood chip mulch. With loose parts, tools, and supplies, children can create art—an exploration of color, form, and texture; or a representation of their lives and the issues they're facing. When children feel in control of their space and materials, they get excited, inspired, and motivated to accomplish things. The sense of mastery that comes from creating something on one's own is invaluable; confidence grows when children feel their impact on their world.

As children work with these components to understand the world, there is often an element of destruction in their play. Sometimes this is rooted in curiosity about cause and effect and the properties of different objects and materials. For instance, they may wonder "What will happen if . . . " as they test the force required to crack or bend something that may seem fragile or rigid. Sometimes there is delight, slapstick humor, or a sense of power that comes with causing mayhem. Sometimes using muscles and exerting force is a helpful way to release tension or frustration or anger. It is important to support these impulses by offering appropriate outlets. There can be fun opportunities to smash sand castles, drop old pumpkins off high places, throw rocks into water, knock things down, and whack things with sticks. All of these need to be paired with emotional support and conversations about respecting things others have made or value as well as living things like fragile plants and animals' homes.

Building

The opposite of the destructive impulse can also be satisfied through play with loose parts—delicate activities that build and balance and create. It is in building that children have the opportunity to nurture and care, to create cozy beds and safe homes for dolls and toy animals and pretend families.

To take full advantage of helping kids build with loose parts, the key is to have many different *kinds* of things and a lot of at least some of the things. Natural materials are ideal for this, both in quantity and diversity. Outfitting your space with loose parts that inspire children to experiment, create, and invent tells them we have faith in their abilities. They begin by envisioning a goal, alone or with friends, then, using the materials at hand, they try, observe what works, revise, refine, and keep testing the results. This is the foundation of the scientific method and it's a type of play that produces problem solvers.

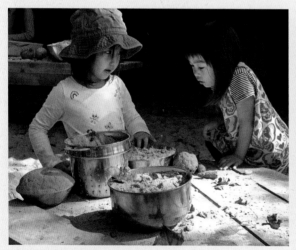

Big sister explains her concoction of sand, leaves, and Osage oranges to little sister.

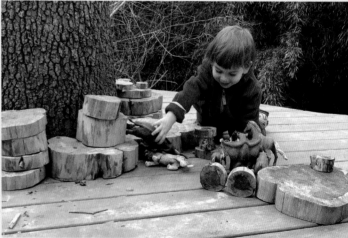

Tree cookies of different sizes paired with rubber animals invite a whole different kind of outdoor play.

An abundance and variety of building materials give permission to experiment, think big, and to develop complexity in planning and execution. At the same time, skills such as tool handling and a knowledge of different materials are being acquired. Young builders learn quickly that rocks make good foundations, sand is malleable, and mud can hold things together. Working together, kids also develop their abilities to communicate, negotiate, and cooperate to come up with solutions.

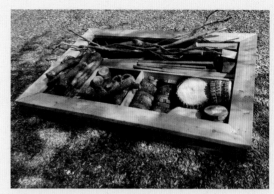

The variety and quantity of loose parts available increases the options for experimenting, makes for flexible thinking, and leads to risk-taking, problem-solving, and self-confidence.

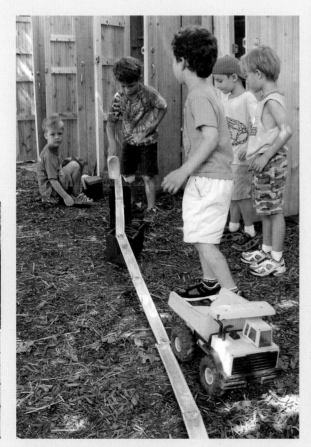

It took a lot of thinking and testing to get the slope right for water to flow down this split bamboo channel.

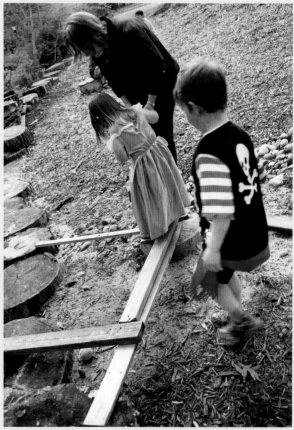

Here, kids arranged the parts, then let family members test their balance.

TYPES OF LOOSE PARTS

A rich selection of loose parts can include both natural and manufactured items, building parts, fasteners, and tools. Real stuff has tremendous play value—especially combined with sand, water, and soil.

NATURAL LOOSE PARTS

* bamboo poles
* curly bark chunks
* cut grasses, weeds, branches
* cypress knees
* dirt clods
* driftwood
* flat stones (to stack)
* flowers
* gnarly logs and burls
* hollow tree sections
* logs and tree cookies of different diameters and thicknesses (from tiny 1 by 1 inch, to too big to lift)
* mud, especially with clayey soil
* old Christmas trees
* seasonal leaves
* shells
* sticks of different lengths, diameters, and bark textures
* stones, pebbles, rocks
* straw bales (tied, cut apart, or as loose straw)
* vines and vine pieces

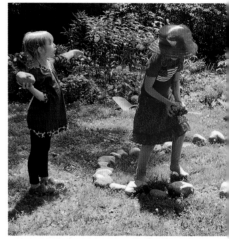

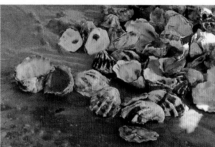

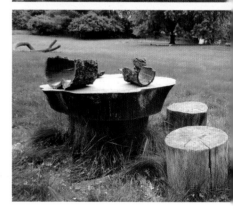

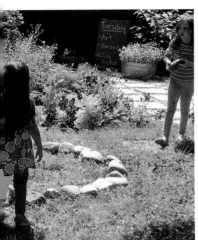

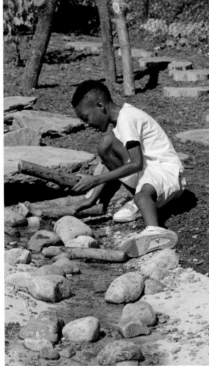

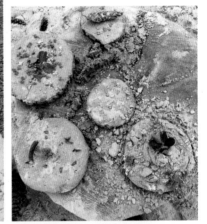

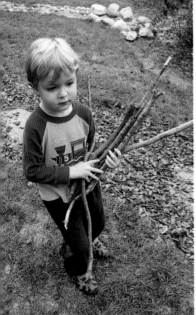

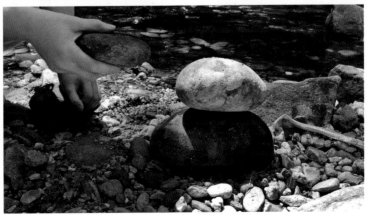

TYPES OF LOOSE PARTS (CONTINUED)

MANUFACTURED LOOSE PARTS

* boards and lumber
* cans, buckets, bins, crates
* cardboard boxes, tubes
* chairs, tables
* dollhouses
* dolls and doll accessories
* dress-up clothes and props (scarves, hats, helmets, crowns, boots, capes, briefcases, suitcases)
* fabric (sheets, blankets, towels, rugs)
* heavy things that require two to lift
* pipes and pipe sections (PVC, corrugated, metal, clear acrylic, hollowed-out bamboo, gutters, downspouts, vacuum cleaner hoses, pieces of garden hose)
* pots, pans, kitchen utensils (especially metal and wood)
* sawhorses
* spools
* steering wheels and tires
* things to take apart, with parts that can be used for creating (broken appliances, cameras, mechanical toys)
* toy animals
* toy vehicles
* wagons, bikes

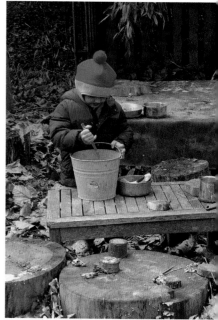

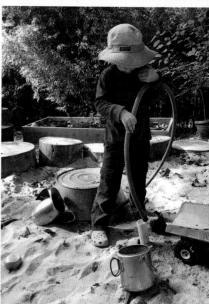

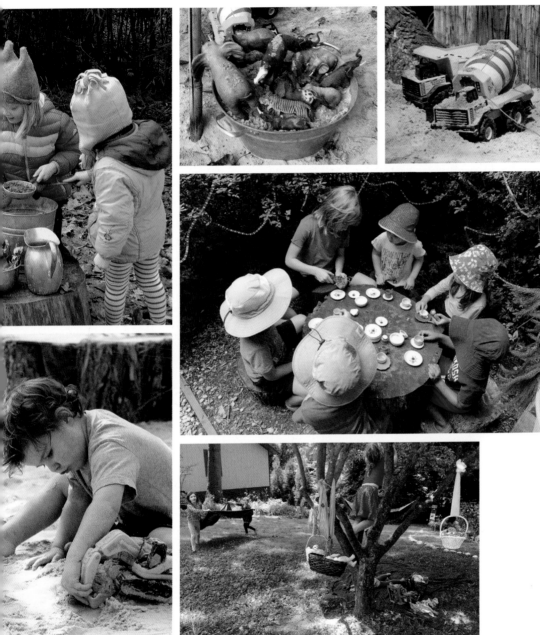

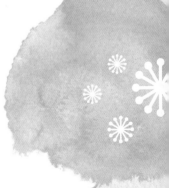

Safe tool use

Teaching children how to use tools safely is important not only because it prevents injuries, but because it increases the chances of success in building things. Using tools like hammers, saws, wrenches, and screwdrivers develops the muscles of the hand, wrist, and arms—all essential for fine motor skills such as writing, drawing, cutting, and painting.

There are stages of learning that begin with the youngest children. For example, babies can hammer wooden pegs into holes. Toddlers can hammer golf tees into the ground. Preschoolers can use real hammers to pound nails into a stump once you set the nails in place. The next stage might be hammering a nail into a board, learning to use a clamp to hold things in place, and then actually building simple wooden assemblies. Sawing begins with using wooden spreaders to cut into butter or soft cheese, then using a real hand saw to cut a block of cardboard held in a clamp. Next might be sawing a piece of wood in a clamp, with an adult spotting.

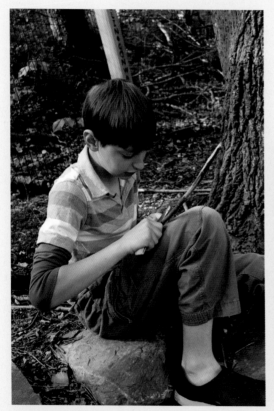

A pocketknife for whittling is an appropriate tool for an older child, but it should come with a lesson in knife safety.

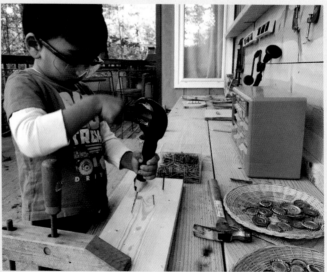

On an outside deck, a simple shelf outfitted with a clamp, board, tools, and hardware becomes an engrossing woodworking station.

ADVENTURE PLAY

A movement to create adventure playgrounds is growing across the United States. Born in 1940s Denmark, the first "junk playgrounds" included all sorts of rubble, along with fire pits, waterways, and even farm animals. The concept spread across Europe to Germany, England, France, the Netherlands, Switzerland, and other parts of Scandinavia. Adventure playgrounds today are child-ruled spaces, often in urban areas, that provide abundant and varied loose parts, building materials, tools, and a limited number of adults—as facilitators, but not usually initiators of activities.

Another model for today's adventure playground is the work yard or junk playground found in Israeli kibbutzim. These children's spaces were stocked with old machinery, vehicles, tools, and other discarded materials. Children who played there were required only to have a current tetanus shot to roam free. The goal was to produce competent, adventurous kids.

The Adventure Playground in Berkeley, California, is the longest continuously running program in the United States. More recently, adventure playgrounds have sprung up from New York to Washington state, in Texas, Nebraska, and other parts of the country.

For more information, check out the North American Adventure Play Association at adventureplayground.org. You may also want to watch *The Land*, a documentary film about a Welsh adventure playground.

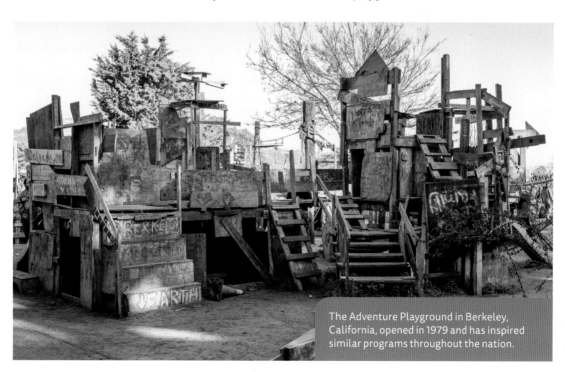

The Adventure Playground in Berkeley, California, opened in 1979 and has inspired similar programs throughout the nation.

PLANT PARTS for PLAY

PLANT TYPE	DESCRIPTION
GRASS	River oats (*Chasmanthium latifolium*). The seeds or oats are dangling jewels, which are great fun to pick. The dense roots make this plant perfect for holding banks and preventing erosion. They also make it difficult to get rid of the plant if you ever change your mind—so plant carefully.
ANNUAL FLOWERS	Zinnias*, cosmos*, marigolds*, and pansies* produce two flowers for every one you pick.
PERENNIAL FLOWERS	Purple coneflower (*Echinacea purpurea*), black-eyed Susan (*Rudbeckia hirta*), tickseed (*Coreopsis* species), obedient plant (*Physostegia virginiana*), and swamp sunflower (*Helianthus angustifolius*) all have abundant flowers to pick.
CONIFER CONES	All coniferous trees produce cones, and all produce male and female cones—sometimes on the same tree, sometimes on separate trees, depending on the species. Conifers with interesting cones for play: hemlock (*Tsuga canadensis*), Douglas fir (*Pseudotsuga menziesii*), bald cypress (*Taxodium distichum*), dawn redwood* (*Metasequoia glyptostroboides*), and eastern red cedar (*Juniperus virginiana*).
TREES WITH PODS	Kentucky coffeetree (*Gymnocladus dioicus*), catalpa (*Catalpa* species), and redbud (*Cercis canadensis*) each have long, sometimes rattling seed pods. Magnolia (*Magnolia grandiflora*) pods are fun to collect (and throw). American sweetgum (*Liquidambar styraciflua*) has prickly round seed pods. *I wouldn't advise planting sweetgum in a space for children, because the pods hurt to step on, but if it's already growing, the prickly spheres are fun to collect and use for art projects.*
ACORNS	Different kinds of oak trees (*Quercus* species) produce acorns of different sizes and shapes.
BERRIES	Beautyberry (*Callicarpa americana*) has beautiful magenta berries that aren't delicious to people but aren't toxic, and birds love them. Bayberry (*Myrica pensylvanica*) produces waxy berries that were used to make scented candles in colonial days. Winterberry (*Ilex verticillata*) is a deciduous holly; plant a male and female to get berries, but don't eat them because they are mildly toxic.

*Indicates non-native. All other plants listed are North American natives.

ART IN THE OUTDOORS

The outdoors can include space and materials for building *and* for art: painting, writing, drawing, sculpting, and making music. From a logistical perspective, outside is often the best place for big, loud, messy, exuberant play. This might include making raucous music or hammering with abandon, sawing wood or working with gloppy paint.

Painting and Drawing

Art in the out-of-doors allows for larger scale and messier work than we might tolerate indoors. There's no need to worry about a mess when hosing off is an easy cleanup option. Paint can be tempera, watercolor, or whatever washable paints you find at your local crafts store. Tools can be fingers or feet, foam or bristle brushes of all sizes, clumps of pine needles, or frayed sticks.

Things to paint on include wood, paper, cardboard, fabric, rocks, mirrors, and oneself. Painting on one's own body is fun (for some

children) and outside it's easy to hose off. (For a tactile-sensitive child, dipping one finger in paint might be a challenge just big enough or perhaps even more than they are comfortable with. Everyone needs to go at their own pace.) Consider different types of horizontal and vertical work surfaces that will support a variety of work styles, body types, energy levels, and motor skills.

Large painting surfaces allow arms to move to their full extension and build core (chest,

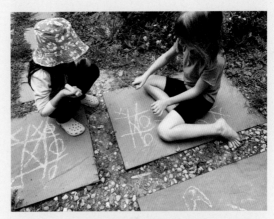

Working on the ground lets children assume a variety of positions: squatting, sitting, sprawling out—whatever works in the moment.

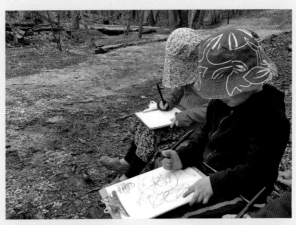

Rocks can be painted and transformed into animals and other figures or used as decorations in the space. Holding onto a slippery, paint-covered rock is a fine motor challenge.

Clipboards support writing and drawing in the field.

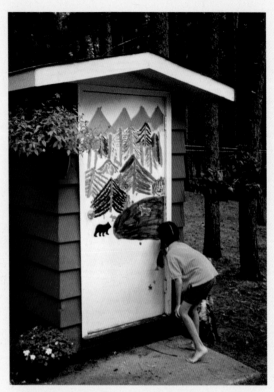

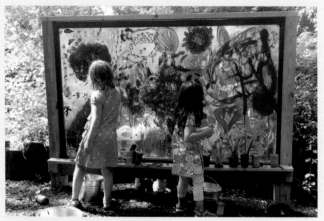

Writing or drawing on a vertical surface uses the muscles of shoulders, elbows, wrists, and hands differently than a horizontal surface and both are important experiences.

Encouraging kids to create a mural on a blank surface such as a shed door communicates respect for them and their work.

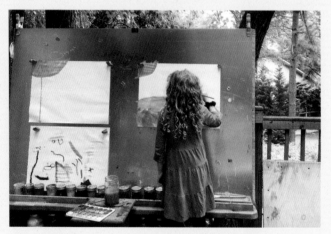

Sheet metal mounted on plywood allows paper to be attached with magnets. On a different day, magnets can be the focus of play.

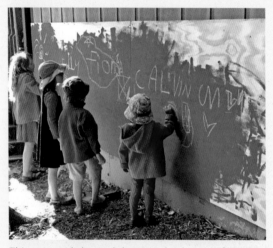

This mounted plywood sheet received a coat of blue paint one day, then was decorated with chalk the next. The large work surface lets children work expansively.

stomach, neck, and back) muscles. Working on a large vertical surface encourages children to reach across their bodies, an important ability to master for smooth and satisfying fine motor actions such as writing and drawing, and also a key task in healthy brain development. This is known as crossing the midline.

Work surfaces of varying heights allow multiple body positions and accommodate a range of motor abilities. Working directly on the ground allows a lot of flexibility and repositioning. Children can squat, sit, or kneel on the ground at a low table, sit on backless benches or stools, or stand at a tall table or vertical surface. There can be slate, stone, and chalkboard surfaces for drawing with chalk or painting with water, frames for building giant mobiles and sculptures, and metal panels for magnets and magnetic poetry. An easel made with a clear acrylic panel and installed so both sides are accessible allows multiple artists to paint interactively. Paper can be attached to the easel, or paint can be applied directly to the acrylic with fingers, brushes, sponges, or other tools. Paper can also be laid over wet paint on the plexiglass to make a print. Or it can be all about process and more ephemeral. When paint covers the view through, the world disappears, but a wet sponge and squeegee help the view beyond reappear and make removing the paint as much fun as applying it.

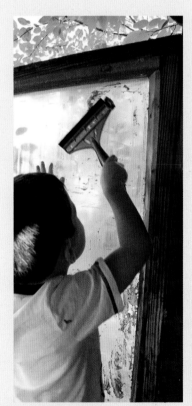

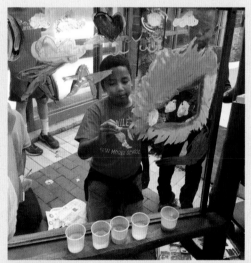

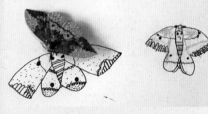

A clear acrylic panel offers a unique perspective on the process of applying paint, for both the artist and the audience.

A determined child scrubs and squeegees dried paint off the clear easel, revealing a view of nature and beautiful light shining through.

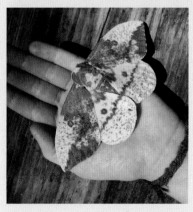

The outdoors is full of creative inspiration. Finding this beautiful butterfly led to a drawing session to capture the wing patterns. Color was then added. Having drawing materials close at hand meant the artist could dive in the moment inspiration hit.

Sculpture

Clay may be dug from the earth if you live in a place with that type of soil, or purchased from an art supply store. Sculpting with clay, or any modeling material, is a soothing, tactile activity that will allow your children to explore creating in three dimensions. Clay tends to be more difficult to mold than softer modeling materials, giving kids more challenge and involving more core strength to manipulate it. Clay is a special type of soil, in that the tiny particles that comprise it make it especially malleable, but it can dry very hard.

With a variety of materials and fasteners (string, wire, glues of different types, paste, yarn, staples, clips, and clamps) kids can also do found-object sculpture. Creations can happen on the ground or on tables, and in the case of mobiles, can hang from branches or overhead wood frames.

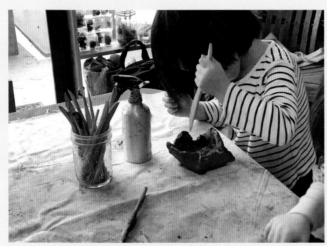

Working with clay is good for developing fine motor control and hand muscles, as well as the ability to use tools for rolling, hammering, scoring, and cutting.

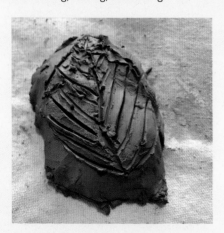

Clay can be molded, flattened, etched, and sliced with hands and tools.

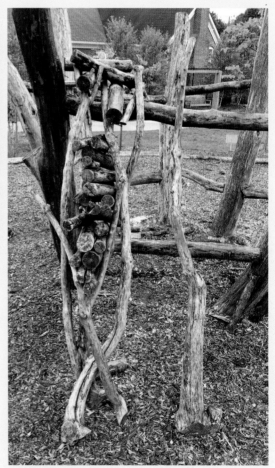

Using only sticks and logs, this delicately balanced arrangement expresses both artfulness and engineering.

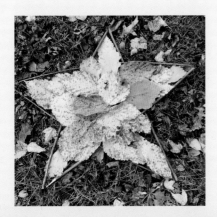

An ephemeral star is made with twigs and colorful leaves.

Weaving

The process of weaving together varied materials and creating patterns is valuable as a stand-alone experience, without a focus on the product. But if children are interested, the weavings they make with natural materials can be dried and displayed as a way to bring nature inside. An outdoor loom can be a small square frame for personal weaving, or large enough for a group to weave together. Either can utilize natural materials like grasses, flower stalks, and branches along with string, ribbon, and yarn woven through a loom warped with twine or string.

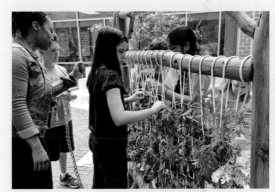

Weaving with others fosters community, and the tapestry that's woven can become a symbol of that community. Earthloom.org offers plans for building an outdoor loom, along with curriculum and their philosophy of building community through weaving as a ceremonial activity.

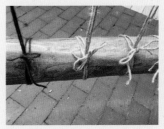

Mark the center with a different colored string. Loop and tie the other end around the bottom bar.

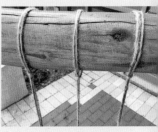

Warp the loom with twine or string by looping doubled string over the top bar.

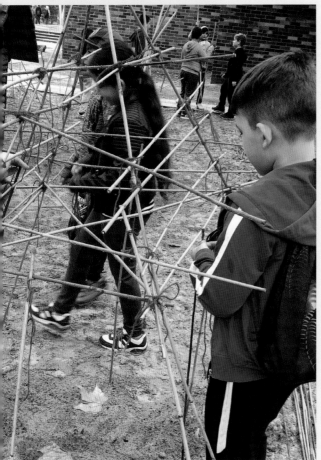

Thin bamboo poles and yarn can inspire a variety of three-dimensional creations.

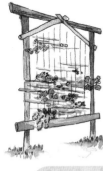

PLANTS FOR WEAVING AND DYEING

For Weaving

PLANT TYPE	PART TO USE
Seasonal blossoms	Flowers on stems can be woven in, even if they aren't long enough to go all the way across.
Sticks and branches such as river birch (*Betula nigra*), **willow, red twig dogwood**	Peeling, shaggy bark
Tall grasses, including little bluestem (*Schizachyrium scoparium*) **and switchgrasses** (*Panicum virgatum*), **especially 'Heavy Metal' cultivar.**	Tall stalks, leaves, and flowers
Tall perennials such as ironweed (*Vernonia noveboracensis*), **goldenrod** (*Solidago species*), **black-eyed Susan** (*Rudbeckia hirta*), **and obedient plant** (*Physostegia virginiana*).	Stems, leaves, and flowers

For Dyeing

DYE COLOR	PLANT TYPES AND PIECES
MAGENTA	Berries of staghorn sumac (*Rhus typhina*), pokeberry (*Phytolacca americana*). (Caution: all parts of pokeberry plant are toxic; do not ingest.)
RED	Blood root (*Sanguinaria canadensis*). Native Americans used its sap as face paint.
ORANGE	Carrot juice, onion skins
YELLOW	Petals of goldenrod (*Solidago*), black-eyed Susan (*Rudbeckia hirta*), or dandelion. Make a dyebath, or pound petals between sheets of cotton.
GREEN	Grass. Rub or hammer grass blades between sheets of cotton.
BLUE/PURPLE	Petals of pansies or violets (*Viola species*). Pound between sheets of cotton. False indigo (*Baptisia australis*). Create a dyebath.
BROWN	Black walnut (*Juglans nigra*). The husks from nuts will dye your skin, and in a dyebath will turn cloth a rich brown. Acorns from oak trees (*Quercus* family) are another source of brown pigment.

All plants listed are North American natives.

The artful yard

Children's art adds character and beauty and a sense of place to any space. Including children's art in a play space communicates the message to them, and to the world, that their work is valued and that this is a space that belongs to the children.

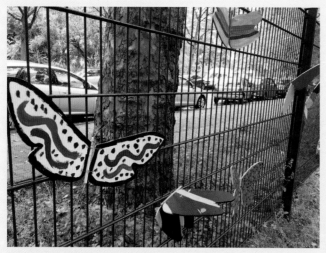

Painted wooden butterflies add whimsical color to a drab fence (see accompanying project).

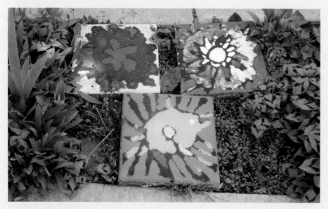

Painted stepping stones provide a shortcut across a garden bed.

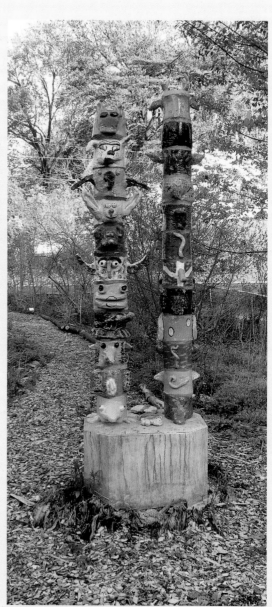

Totem art made of clay faces marks the entry to the walking trail adjacent to a play space.

BUTTERFLY CUTOUTS

Children can be in charge of the drawing and painting portions of this project, and possibly the cutting, depending on age. This technique can also be used to cut and paint other shapes such as flowers out of wood.

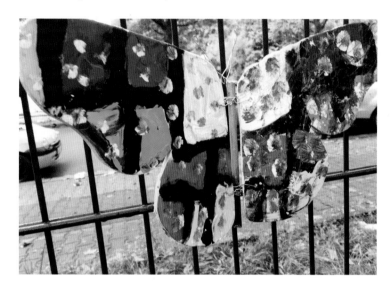

WHAT YOU'LL NEED

* drawing paper
* scissors
* outline of a butterfly wing
* two small wood panels, ⅛ to ¼ inch thick
* wooden dowel or stick
* hand saw or utility knife, depending on board thickness
* drill
* water-based outdoor craft paint and brushes
* clear paint sealant
* craft wire

1 Draw the outline of one butterfly wing on a piece of paper.

2 Cut out a pattern, following the outline.

3 Using the pattern, trace one outline onto a piece of wood, then flip the pattern to trace the mirror image of the opposite wing on the other wood panel.

4 Cut the wings from the wood with a hand saw or utility knife, depending on the thickness of the wood.

5 Drill two or three holes along the inside edges of both wings.

6 Paint the wings as symmetrically as desired, one side at a time, letting each wing dry before flipping to paint the back.

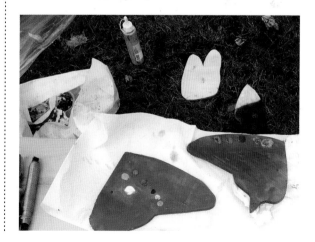

7 Paint a section of wooden dowel or a stick for the body.

8 Cover all the painted surfaces with clear sealant.

9 Fasten the wings to the body with wire and use more wire to form antennae.

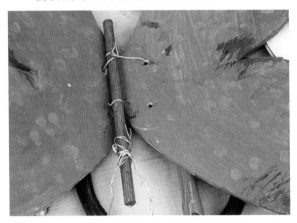

10 Artfully attach your butterfly to a fence.

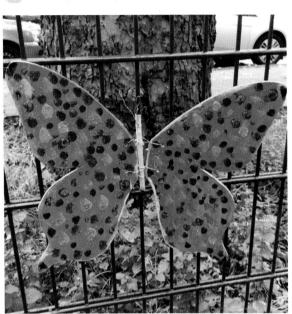

11 Create a butterfly fence by adding an entire flock.

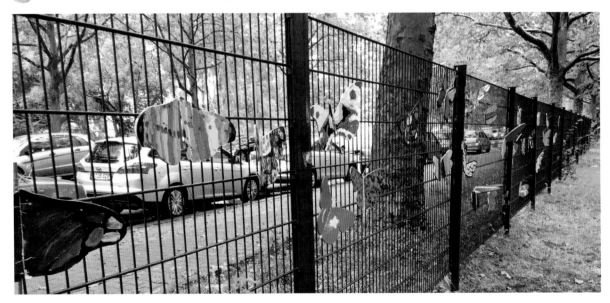

WHERE TO STORE IT ALL

Having loose parts in a play space is all well and good, but where do those parts live between play times? Storage can take many forms, from small bins to big sheds and everything in between. Shallow cabinets that are one bin deep make the contents easy to access, unlike deep sheds where things can get lost. Closed storage, where materials can be secured behind doors, creates less visual clutter. Open storage lets the items stored stay visible and could include shelves, hooks, and clear or open bins. Storage containers can be baskets and bins of varied sizes made of natural materials or plastic.

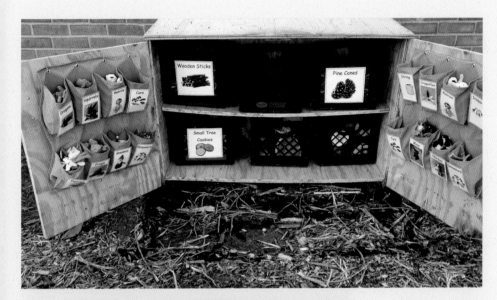

Labels and pictures on storage containers help young kids with language and visual identification.

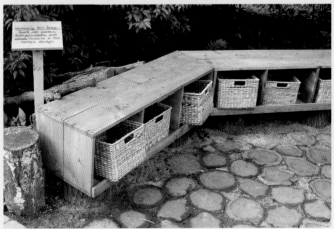

Baskets and bins keep toys and loose parts organized.

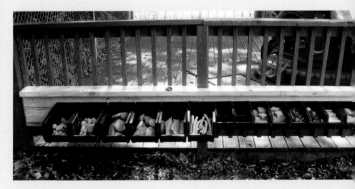

Aesthetically, the space will feel calmer if storage containers are uniform sizes and in a limited range of colors and materials. Think about a convenient way to store each unique category of items: sticks in a tall rack or barrel, a hook for hoops and other odd-shaped items, garden tools in an old mailbox near where they are used. Organized storage is key because it allows children to know where to find things the things they need. A predictable environment is calming and helps children feel secure. Labeling every hook, bin, shelf, and cabinet makes it simple to find what you need when you need it, and more likely that things will be put away. It can be as simple as permanent marker on a plastic bin, or a laminated photo of whatever goes inside, to allow a pre-reader to find what is needed and be in charge of storing it when play time is over.

Where possible, create point-of-use storage, where materials are kept close to where they are used. Consider ways that children of varying mobility can access what they need, whether that means at a height that is easy to reach, or with fasteners and latches that can be easily maneuvered. Conversely, for things that need to be under adult control, use height and latched doors as a way to limit access.

In order to keep the space manageable for adults and not overwhelming to children, it may be helpful to limit what is available at any one time. Loose parts need to change over time to keep things interesting. One role of adults in the space is to replenish, rotate materials, and introduce new supplies and tools that are responsive to children's interests and developmental stages. Storage makes all of this possible.

Think about the way materials are displayed. Monitor the quantity of pieces in closed versus open storage. For younger children especially, it is important that adults help manage loose parts, so that the number displayed is not visually or cognitively overwhelming. Create thoughtfully displayed arrangements of toys and materials to invite children to play and perhaps to use materials in new ways.

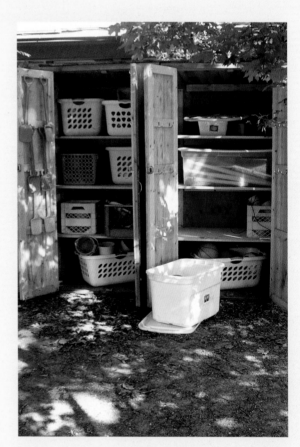

Shallow cabinets stocked with bins help children find toys quickly—and put them away, when it's time.

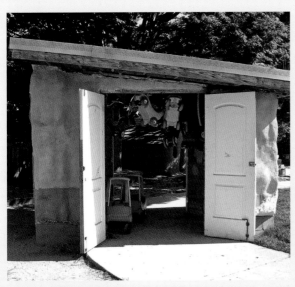

A shunnel (shed plus tunnel) is a multi-purpose shed outfitted with doors on opposite ends.

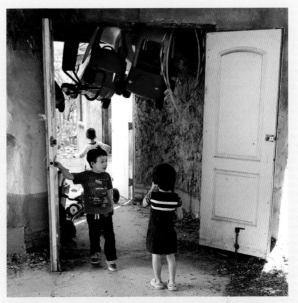

During play, the shunnel's doors are open, allowing a fun pass-through for trike riders and walkers. Later, bikes and wagons can be stored inside and the doors latched.

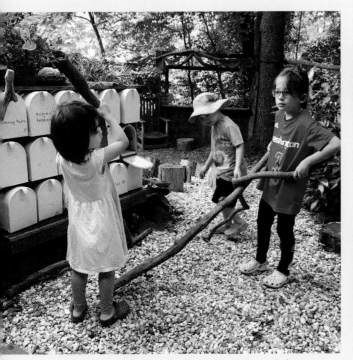

A bank of mailboxes works for both storage and play.

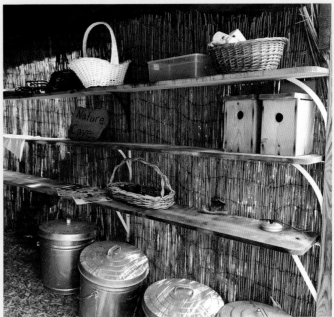

If there's room, consider using space under the deck for storage.

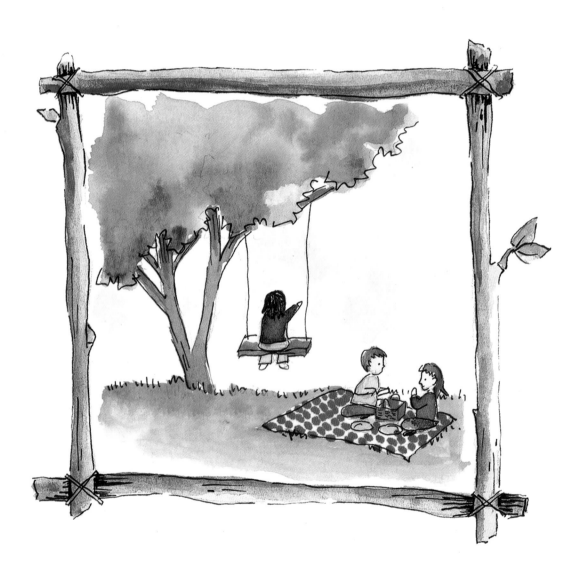

CREATING COMFORT

"What is needed is planned complexity:
an environment rich enough to challenge
but not so complex as to be frustrating."

—from *Caring Spaces, Learning Places:*
Children's Environments that Work, by Jim Greenman

An inviting and comfortable outdoor space will pull your family out of the house. If your space is designed to meet everyone's needs for shelter, shade, play, and places to gather, children and adults will be happy outside and more likely to spend time there.

SHELTER

Porches and covered transition spaces connect indoors and out, and provide shelter from the elements. Part house, part outdoor space, a porch is protected, yet with fresh air and clear sounds of nature. It is a place where one feels sheltered, but with a little added freedom. On the porch, it's okay to eat and spill, to splash water, or to paint more exuberantly than indoors. It is also a place where we might feel relaxed enough to read, nap, maybe even sleep for the whole night. The pace of life feels slower and more relaxed here. Porches connect us to life in the neighborhood from a safe vantage point, in a space that is clearly ours. In powerful ways, time on a porch soothes our souls.

There are also uncovered transition spaces, such as decks and patios, that are directly connected to the house. These allow inside activities to spill out to an open space that is less wild than the garden, but where the connection to nature begins to infuse our experience.

Finally, there are freestanding outdoor shelters, roofed structures like gazebos and pavilions, where we are protected from the rain and sun, yet we can enjoy the sounds of birds and the feeling of breezes. These structures can be anywhere in the landscape, bringing shelter to more remote places, or overlooking a beautiful view.

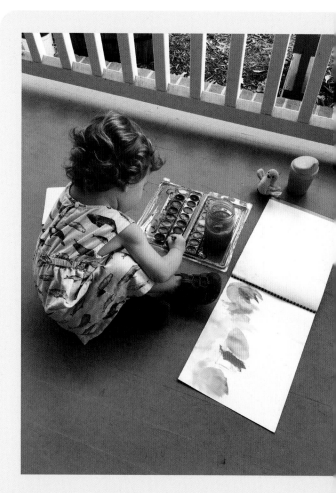

A porch with books and art materials plus a space to sit and work brings indoor activities out. But porches can also be places to just watch the weather and seasons change from a protected spot.

Porches and gazebos can have open sides, or they may have screens to protect us from stinging and annoying insects. In certain buggy parts of the country, screens are what make the difference between being able to relax outside for an extended period or not. Without exception, every client of mine who has added a screened porch has said that it changed their life and their family's relationship to the yard. It allows them to be outside in comfort for large portions of the day (and night), for at least part of the year.

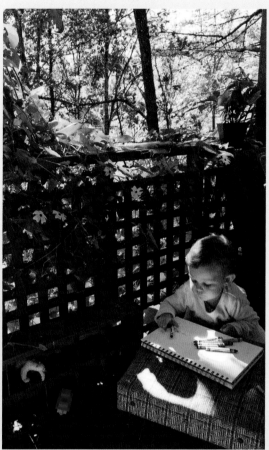

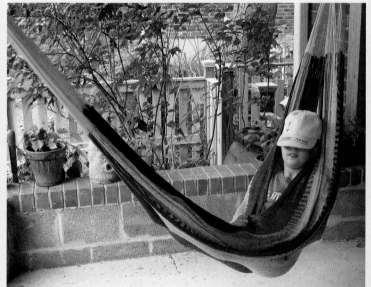

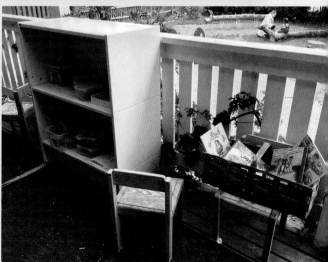

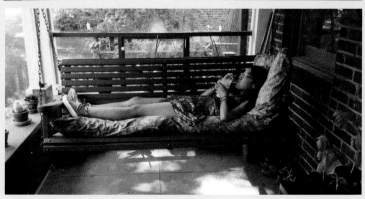

SHADE

Before there was air conditioning, shade was what made it comfortable to be outside in hot weather. Shade protects our skin from the dangers of overexposure to sun and helps make it safe to be outside.

Shade can be created by the ceiling of an outdoor room. It can be creative and interesting and playful. Fabric shade sails are a way to quickly and affordably add softness, color, and sun protection to a space. They can be anchored to trees, posts, or to a building. Shadows can add texture, patterns, and even educational content to the space through creative cutouts in arbors, lattice, or woven bamboo mats that make interesting shade patterns. A trellis, pergola, or arbor planted with deciduous vines will provide lush, cooling shade in the growing season, and when the leaves fall in the autumn, the sunshine you crave will be there to warm you.

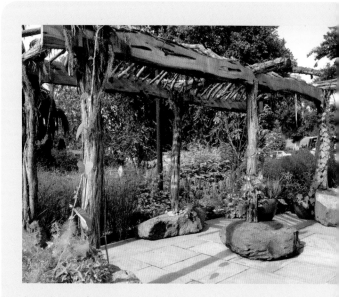

A rustic pergola is set on boulders.

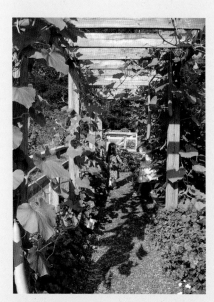

Veggies are easy to access growing down from this arbor.

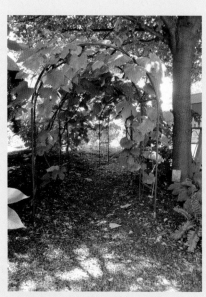

A tunnel's overhead vines create greenery and shade.

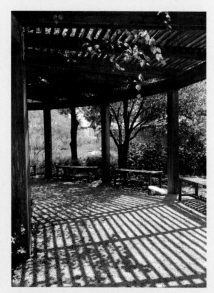

A pergola creates beautiful shadow patterns at Lady Bird Johnson Wildflower Center.

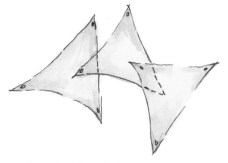

PROJECT

POSTS AND SHADE SAILS

WHAT YOU'LL NEED

* shade sails (available from many sources online in a variety of shapes, sizes, and colors)
* tape measure
* shovel
* gravel for bottom of post holes (enough to fill the bottom 4 to 6 inches of each post hole)
* pressure-treated wood posts, or locust posts with bark removed (3 posts for one shade sail; for more than one sail, draw the arrangement in advance so you can see how many adjacent corners of sails can share a post, and to calculate how many posts you'll need)

* 2-by-4-inch boards, hammer, nails (for stabilizing posts)
* ready-mix concrete (enough to fill each post hole from the top of the gravel)
* wheelbarrow or basin for mixing concrete
* water source
* drill
* hardware: one eye bolt and one turnbuckle for each shade sail corner
* pliers

---

1 Lay the shade sails on the ground and create a pleasing arrangement. It's nice to have them overlap to create unbroken shade. You can mount them at different heights for visual interest.

2 Once you have an arrangement, measure 6 inches beyond the end of the shade sails and mark that as the location of the edge of the post, adding half the diameter of the post to determine the center of the hole.

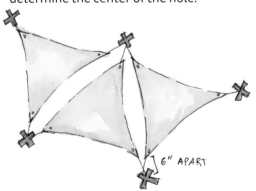

6" APART

3 Dig the post holes to 2 feet deep, or whatever the frost depth is in your area.

2' DEEP

4-6" GRAVEL

FROST LINE

4 Pour 4 to 6 inches of gravel into the bottom of the post hole.

5 Set the post on top of the gravel, be sure it's level, and temporarily secure it with 2-by-4-inch board braces.

2 × 4

6 Mix and add concrete on top of gravel in the hole, until concrete is even with ground. Let concrete set.

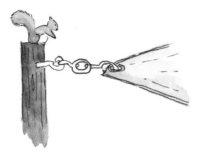

7 Remove temporary braces once concrete has set.

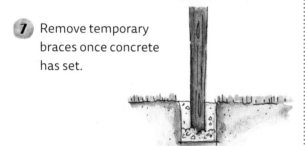

8 Drill holes for eye bolts on the appropriate side of the posts. Be sure to locate the eyes bolts so the finished sail will be angled to let rainwater run off.

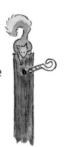

9 Fasten the sails to the eye bolts using turn-buckles through the grommet holes in the shade sails.

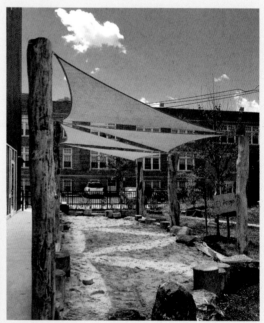

10 Tighten the cable until the shade sails are taut.

11 Relax in the shade!

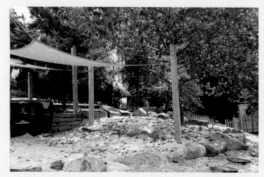

Shade sails make both of these sandpits cool oases for play on a hot day.

Trees as shade

Trees are the most straightforward, long-lasting, and relatively effortless way to access the shade we all need. The pool of shade beneath a tree, especially on a hot day, can be very inviting. If there is a beautiful tree in your space, think about enhancing it to become a play or gathering destination. An invitation can be as simple as adding a picnic table underneath, a bench around the trunk, or even something as subtle as a circle of stones a few feet out from the trunk. It may not look like much to adults, but this simple outline creates a space that calls to children. If enhanced with toys or loose parts, it will inspire imagination.

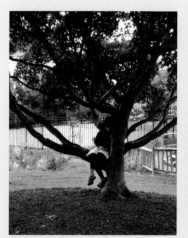

A girl, a book, and a seat in a tree.

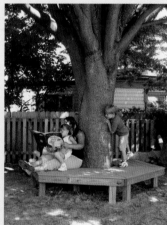

This trunk-encircling platform is extra deep for seating and play.

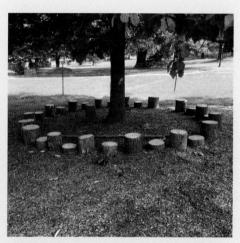

A circle of stumps in the shade can be used for many purposes.

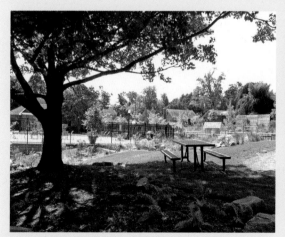

A picnic table in the shade offers a cool respite.

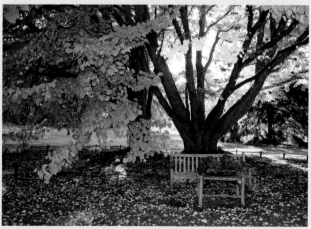

Benches under trees encourage sitting for a spell and soaking up nature.

Shade Trees: An Investment in the Future

Planting a tree, especially one we hope will grow big enough to shade our yards generously, is not an act that will return benefits quickly. It is a gift to our children and all who come after us. It is an act of faith.

American hophornbeam (*Ostrya virginiana*) Features a rounded crown and spread of 25 to 30 feet.

American linden (*Tilia americana*) Fragrant, pale yellow flowers in spring attract honeybees and other pollinators, and can also be made into tea.

Maple (*Acer* species) Sugar maple (*Acer saccharum*) and red maple (*Acer rubrum*) provide spreading branches and great fall color.

Musclewood (*Carpinus caroliniana*) Known for smooth, beautiful bark that resembles muscles.

Redbud (*Cercis canadensis*) Look for yellow fall color and edible purple flowers in spring.

Swamp white oak (*Quercus bicolor*) Medium-sized tree with large glossy leaves.

Thornless honey locust (*Gleditsia triacanthos* var. *inermis*) A fast-growing tree with tiny leaflets that provide soft, dappled shade and brilliant yellow fall color.

Tulip poplar (*Liriodendron tulipifera*) Spring brings beautiful yellow-orange flowers to this very tall tree.

Tupelo (*Nyssa sylvatica*) Offers beautiful fall color. Honeybees love the flowers.

White oak (*Quercus alba*) The grandest of oaks.

All plants listed are North American natives.

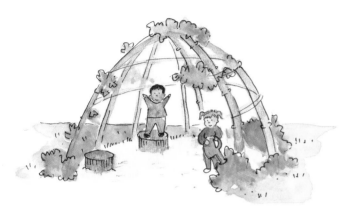

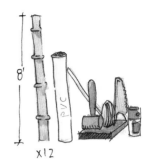

PROJECT

A BAMBOO BOWER

WHAT YOU'LL NEED

* stake
* string
* measuring tape
* landscape-marking spray paint
* 60 inches of PVC pipe, inside diameter a little larger than outside bamboo diameter at its widest
* sledge hammer
* small block of wood
* 12 bamboo poles, each 8 feet long
* 50 plastic cable ties in neutral color
* hand saw
* rust-proof galvanized wire or heavy-duty twine

1. For a 6-foot-diameter bower, choose a location, find the center point, pound the stake into the center point and tie a string to the stake. Measure string 3 feet from the center and mark a 6-foot diameter circle with spray paint.

2. Mark a second circle outside the original circle, 6 inches bigger.

3. Remove any grass and loosen the soil in that 6-inch-wide perimeter ring.

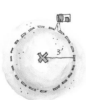 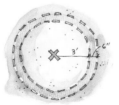

4. Cut the PVC into 6-inch lengths.

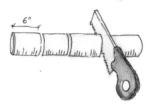

5. Pound the PVC into the ground with a sledge hammer, using the block of wood to protect the PVC from cracking. Space the PVC evenly around the inside edge of the soil circle, leaving an opening for the door.

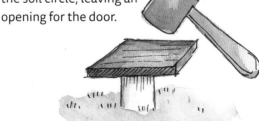

6 Drop the fat end of a bamboo pole into each PVC sleeve.

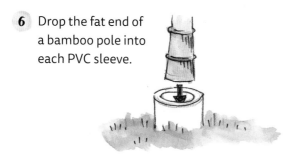

7 Bend opposite poles toward each other to make an arch, overlap the skinny ends of the poles at least 1 foot, and lash them together using wire, twine, or plastic cable ties.

8 Continue around the circle until all poles are

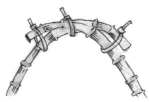

bent into overlapping arches and you have the frame of your bower. You can reinforce the center joint where all the arches cross using rust-proof galvanized wire or heavy-duty twine.

9 Use additional, thinner bamboo poles to make cross pieces, lashing those onto the vertical poles with more cable ties.

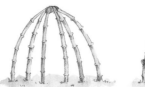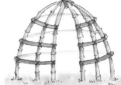

10 Plant a vining plant in the 6-inch strip around the perimeter. See the list of accompanying suggestions.

11 Add a few stumps for seating and a carpet of straw or wood chips, or a blanket, inside the bower.

12 Remember to water the vining plants and guide them to grow up the bamboo poles.

13 This will provide a shady retreat for several years. If you need to replace a pole, it's easy to cut the cable ties, pop the pole out of the PVC sleeve, and insert a new one.

If quick shade is what you need, vines—especially annual vines—are fast growing and a fun, colorful, and sometimes edible way to get coverage. You'll need a structure for the vines to grow on, which can be as simple as a bower or posts set in the ground and connected by wire, or as fancy as an intricate pergola. Plant edible vines over an arch or tunnel, or covering a bamboo shelter frame. The fruits will hang down for easy picking. Vines are also great for covering an unsightly fence or for providing privacy on a porch or deck. Once the structure is in place, get those seeds in the ground!

VINES FOR SHADE, EDIBLES, AND WILDLIFE

PLANT	DESCRIPTION
ANNUAL VINES WITH PROLIFIC FLOWERS	
Black-eye Susan vine*	Yellow-, orange-, or white-petaled flowers have black centers.
Cardinal flower vine*	Provides soft, feathery leaves plus red flowers that attract hummingbirds.
Morning glory*	Sky-blue flowers open in the morning and close by afternoon.
Moonvine*	Giant white flowers open at night and attract pollinating moths.
Cup and saucer vine*	Purple, honey-scented "cups" sit on a green saucer in this fast-growing vine.
Mini pumpkin*	One yellow-flowered vine will produce dozens of tiny orange pumpkins just in time for Halloween.
Decorative gourd*	Can be harvested, dried, and turned into birdhouses (look for selections called "birdhouse" gourds).
PERENNIAL VINES	
Pipevine	Pipevine butterflies lay their eggs on the leaves, so that caterpillars will have a ready source of their favorite food: pipevine leaves. Flowers are greenish purple curved tubes, shaped like a pipe.
Trumpet creeper	Yellow and orange flowers in summer attract hummingbirds and butterflies.
Crossvine	This evergreen vine has beautiful orange flowers in late spring. The woody framework often attracts nesting birds.
Honeysuckle (*Lonicera sempervirens*)	Not the extremely invasive Japanese honeysuckle that is choking many North American hedges and forests. This is a native that comes with pink and yellow or red flowers. Red flowers are a hummingbird magnet.
VINES WITH EDIBLE FRUIT	
Hyacinth bean vine*	Offers gorgeous purple flowers and edible brilliant magenta bean pods.
Scarlet runner bean vine*	Look for fluorescent red flowers. Harvest edible green pods when they are young or wait for the striped beans inside to mature.
Cucumbers*	Plant in the ground and train the vine upward over a trellis. The cucumbers will hang down for easy picking.
Cherry tomatoes*	Will need to be tied up to a frame; can grow to be 8 feet tall or more. The year I grew these on my front arbor I got to grab a snack every time I left the house!

*Indicates non-native. All other plants listed are North American natives.

SEATING

It's certainly possible to sit on the ground, but providing places to perch, sprawl, rock, and relax signal to children (and adults) that this is a place to stay awhile, which is an important message for your outdoor space to communicate. If there are a variety of seating options, the space can meet a range of needs. Include stationary log benches and stump seats along with rockers, swings, hammocks, and gliders that meet different needs for motion.

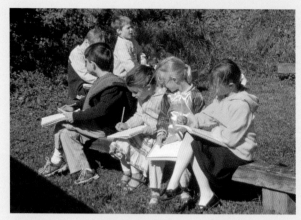

Simple timber benches made of boards are easy to install anywhere.

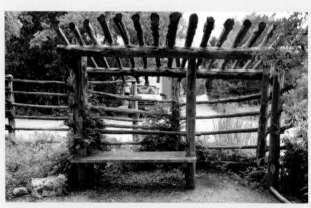

Look for or build rustic benches to carry a nature theme through your yard.

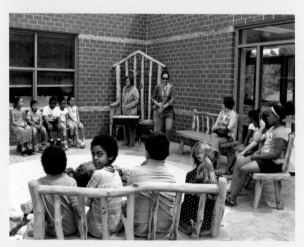

At the Reading Garden at the Drew Model School, this is called the story circle. It includes a giant chair for the storyteller.

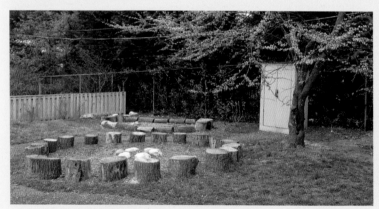

For group seating, consider a circle of logs, stumps, benches, or boulders. This kind of council ring might be just the thing in a favorite backyard where neighborhood children gather.

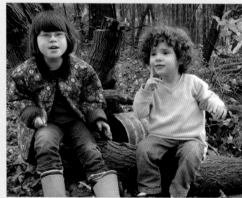

Logs are just the right height for small legs to sit on and take a rest.

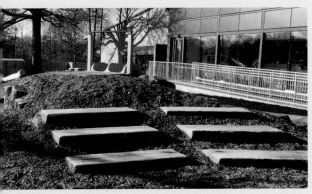

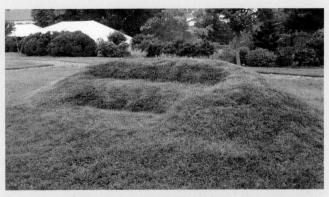

Split logs set into a hillside serve as steps and amphitheater seating.

Lawn Chair is a sofa sculpted of earth and planted with turf at River Farm, headquarters of the American Horticultural Society in Virginia.

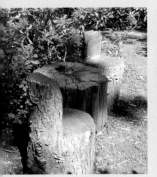

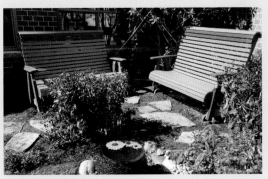

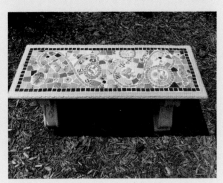

Carved stump seats are easily made with a chainsaw.

Seating placed at right angles encourages conversation.

A mosaic bench made by kids is beautiful and fun to sit on and examine.

Varying the height of seats and having some with backs and some without provides comfort to people of different ages and abilities. A variety of low seating should be available just for children—from single seats for a clearly defined space of one's own, to a bench that can bring together a group. Seating that lets parents rest comfortably and watch and be available to respond to children of different ages and abilities is key. Nearby and low seating is best when outside with a crawling baby or a toddler; seating can be within sight of a 3-year-old. Adults stationed someplace in the vicinity will allow older kids the independence to check in only if needed.

Seating for children and adults together allows for conversation, shared observations, and story reading. When seats are set at right angles to each other, rather than facing each other directly, conversations happen more comfortably. The right-angle arrangement allows eye contact when you want it, but also makes it easy to look away—especially helpful for kids who need some social buffers. If children are distracted and restless when seated with a group, consider that sitting with one's back exposed can trigger a sense of vulnerability. Try letting distracted kids lean against something.

Rockers, swinging chairs and benches, hammocks, gliders, plus all types of swings provide swaying, rocking, and bouncing movement, otherwise known as vestibular stimulation—an experience we all need and find soothing. That sort of motion helps children to understand and sense where their body is in space and to develop a sense of balance. A swinging bench or porch swing is an option that allows children and adults to sit together, or a group of children to share the experience of swinging.

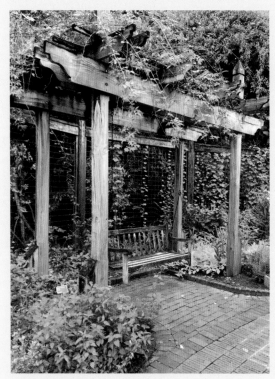

Swings with built-in shade structures are popular with kids and adults alike.

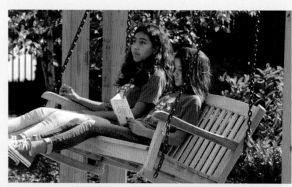

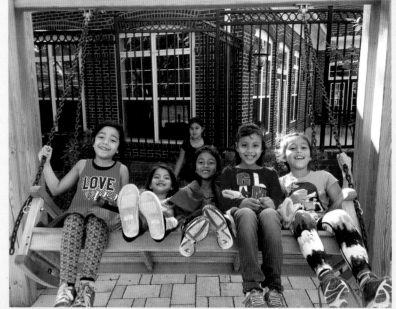

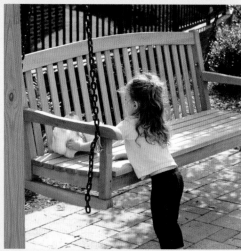

Bench swings are versatile and popular pieces for outdoor spaces, because they meet varied needs: reading and quiet time, imaginative play time, and time with friends.

Hammocks provide soothing rocking motion, along with the softness and responsiveness of fabric. They allow us to lie down and thus invite total relaxation. And yet, with a friend to push you, a ride in a hammock can be a wild adventure. A hammock can be the perfect place for time alone, or with a friend if there's room, or for mom and baby to relax together.

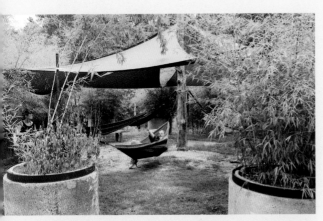

Hammock heaven: a shared post in the center, shade sails, and pots of bamboo around the outer posts.

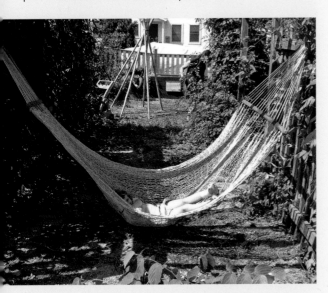

Hammocks can be suspended by anchors other than trees, such as a fence or arbor post, or a large shrub.

WORK SURFACES

Work surfaces facilitate comfortable and extended engagement. The height and orientation can vary to support different positions—standing, sitting, or kneeling—depending on the activity and individual preferences.

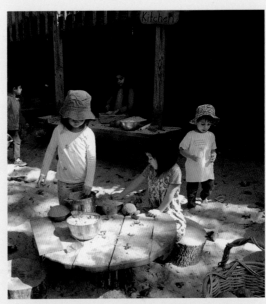

Consider adding work surfaces of different heights. Here a short table in the sandpit lets children work while seated, while a taller surface in the background caters to kids who want to stand.

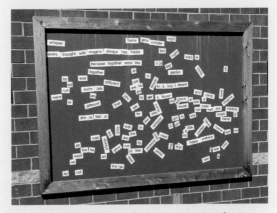

Creative areas should also include vertical surfaces, such as chalkboards, magnet boards, and easels.

WATER SOURCES

Consider easy access to water when locating water-dependent elements of your play space. A rain barrel near the garden will make watering easier and thus more likely to happen. Placing the mud kitchen near a hose bib helps with mixing mud and also makes cleanup more convenient. An outdoor sink does not have to be plumbed in; it can simply be connected to a spigot via PVC pipes. This will simplify rinsing hands, vegetables, and paintbrushes.

A source of drinking water outside, whether from a spigot or a thermos, is essential, especially on a hot day. Only use hoses specially labeled as lead-free for drinking water.

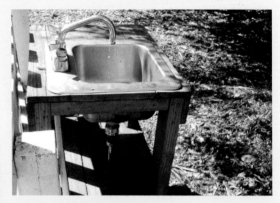

Full plumbing is nice but not essential.

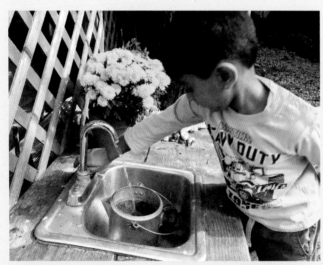

Outdoor sinks come in a variety of styles and ways of working.

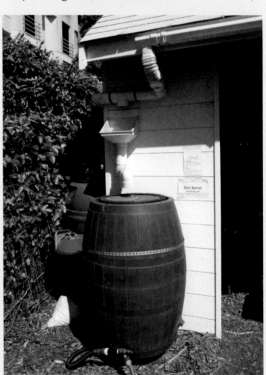

A rain barrel catches roof water for the garden and for play. Standing water can harbor bacteria, so be sure to empty your rain barrel regularly.

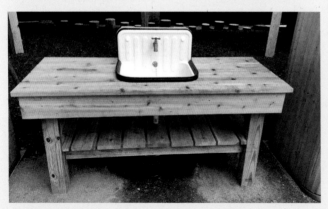

PVC pipes can simply connect the sink to an outdoor spigot.

"THERE'S NO SUCH THING AS BAD WEATHER, ONLY BAD CLOTHING."

This Scandinavian folk saying is a wonderful approach to not letting inclement weather keep us indoors (except in extreme cases, of course). Clothes and gear that respond to the weather are important keys to outdoor comfort. Waterproof pants, boots, hats, and jackets protect children from getting wet when it rains. Plus, pants and boots can be worn anytime to allow kids to play with abandon in water and mud. In the summer, kids need sunblock as well as hats that shelter faces from direct sun. Children's clothing is available that blocks exposure from UV rays, protecting tender skin. Additionally, clothing impregnated with insect repellant helps avoid the toxicity of insecticides applied directly to skin. And, of course, cold weather gear that includes layers, warm gloves or mittens, hats, warm jackets, and snow pants allows kids to savor the magic of winter without getting chilly.

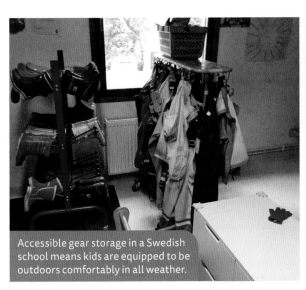

Accessible gear storage in a Swedish school means kids are equipped to be outdoors comfortably in all weather.

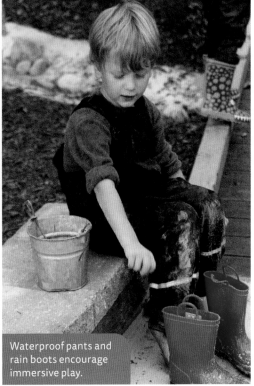

Waterproof pants and rain boots encourage immersive play.

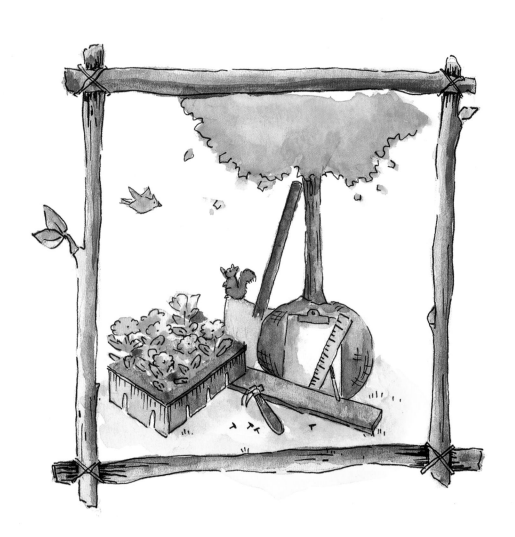

TAKING ACTION

"Dream big. Start small. Don't stop."

—from *Natural Playscapes*, by Rusty Keeler

So here we are. You've digested the previous chapters, or perhaps just perused the photos. Either way, hopefully you're brimming with ideas about what you and your children would like in the play space you're imagining. How do you take all those great ideas and translate them into an actual play space? In this final chapter we will look at ways to fit play into the landscape and make it engaging—and even beautiful.

It almost goes without saying that it's important for kids to have an active role in creating their play space. It is quite possible for children to be involved in every step of the process, or even, depending on the child, for them to own the whole process of creating their nature place. Being mindful of this is key to the success of the space, because kids' involvement means the play space is at least partly their project, and when it's their project, they're more likely to get outside and play.

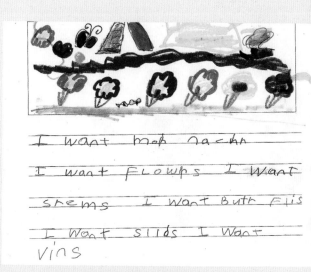

I want moh naahn
I want FLOWPS I want
srems I want Butr Flis
I Wont slids I Want
vins

Even young kids know what they want when they play outside.

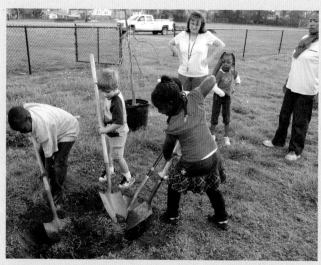

Children can and should have an active role in, and responsibility for, creating their play space—from dreaming to building.

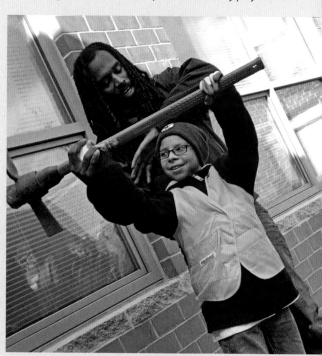

The agency that comes from making decisions and using muscles to make things happen can carry over to confidence in other parts of life.

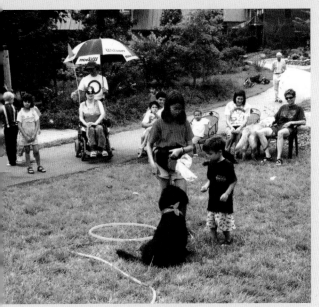

A community dog show was held on the lawn of the common house in our cohousing community. Pedestrian pathways can be seen in the background. Open space for everyone led to many uses beyond play.

GETTING STARTED

When undertaking any project, it usually makes sense to start small and keep things manageable. For example, it might work best, because of how or where you live, to make this a project for your family in your own backyard. On the other hand, you might find it more fun and doable to work together with like-minded others to create your play space. A bigger group of families and stakeholders who are invested in this idea of reconnecting kids to nature will mean the work and cost of building and maintaining a space can be shared. As you build a play area together, you will also build a community, and your children will have friends to play with.

If homes are situated adjacent or nearby, consider pooling backyard space and creating a nature play corridor. This is similar to the concept of a wildlife habitat corridor, in which many property owners near each other in a neighborhood or community plant native plants. This contiguous habitat provides crucial roaming and living space. We can do the same for natural play spaces. If backyards and community common spaces and schoolyards and parks are linked in nature play corridors, children will have more variety in their play settings and are more likely to connect with the critical mass of kids necessary to make play complex, fun, and truly child directed.

My family lived in a cohousing community for many years when my children were young. Cohousing is a model of intentional living that builds community through the design of the houses and the neighborhood. Each household in our community had its own home and small piece of land, but we shared many amenities, including woods, trails, a playing field, a pond, pedestrian pathways between all the houses, and a playground, built by kids and parents using mostly recycled stuff. Without much effort, having this shared land led to lots of unscheduled, unstructured outdoor play by children of all ages, sometimes together, sometimes in small groups, sometimes alone.

I believe that by working together, opening up yards, and agreeing to give children the essential ingredient of *time to play*, families can make this happen in nearly any neighborhood. There are three big steps in the process: **designing**, **funding**, and **building**; each one is made up of lots of little steps. You'll need to come up with a design that works with the site and for the people who are going to use it. You'll need to figure out how much it will cost and where the money will come from. And you'll need to decide how to get it built.

Site Inventory

Use the following to guide your observations. Make notes. Take photos.

* Take in the whole space. Where are the edges? If there is a fence, the edge is clear; if not, what defines the space you're looking at? Notice the shape. Is it square, long and narrow, or irregular? Are there little niches and corners? Is the space adjacent to a house or building?

* Is the space sheltered? Enclosed by landforms, vegetation, buildings? Or open?

* Notice how one gets to the space, the exits, and entries (doors from buildings, gates in the fence, paths leading in).

* Examine the terrain. Flat or sloped? High spots that provide a view, or low spots that feel protected?

* Assess the soil and geology. Is the soil rocky, sandy, clayey? Are there stone outcroppings?

* What is the vegetation? Take note of trees (particularly special or problem ones), shrubs, grasses, perennials, lawn, underbrush, thorns. It is dense or open?

* Are there fixed features such as outbuildings, walkways, or play equipment that are staying or that you want to remove?

* Pay attention to the sun and shade from trees and buildings. This may mean observing at different times of day and in different seasons to get an accurate sense of where your sunny and shady areas are.

* If there are windows that overlook the space, notice what the views are.

* Also pay attention to views looking out of the space and think about framing the best views and screening what is unpleasant, loud, or dangerous.

* Locate water sources. Where do downspouts drain? Where are the hose bibs?

* Check to see where rain goes. Is there a slope into or going away from the space? Are there depressions where puddles form?

* Are there hazards that need to be addressed?

* Are there other assets or problems in the space you want to note?

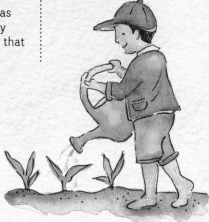

DESIGNING YOUR PLAY SPACE

The first step, creating a design, is a balance. You need to understand your *space*: figure out what it offers and what it needs to work. And you need to understand the *people* who will use that space and what they want and need.

Understanding what you have

We begin by opening our eyes. One essential piece of the foundation of a good design is to really know your site and what is there. Understanding your site requires observing carefully and documenting some information. You may feel as though you know this space like the back of your hand, because, after all, it may be your own backyard. But it's worth it to spend some time examining in a systematic way. Designers call this site inventory. Begin by walking the site, alone or with your children, and really noticing what is good and what is challenging.

This inventory can also be the first aspect of documenting your project from start to finish. Take photos and videos, save pieces from every stage, and if you are so inclined, keep a journal of the process. It will be a wonderful testament to the value of dedication and hard work for both you and your children to look back on—a learning process all its own.

To help remember the space when you're not in it, and to get some objectivity about a place that might be very familiar, take photos. Somehow, looking at the space in a photo gives a new perspective. One technique is to reverse the photo because although it will have the same qualities, it won't look like your space. Seeing through fresh eyes might just open up some new understandings and possibilities.

You'll want to be very clear about where the boundaries of your site are. Sometimes it is easy to ascertain, but it may take some research. You might have to seek out documents like the property plat from your local jurisdiction, site plans from past construction, or surveys from mortgage records to inform this step. There may be stone or metal markers, sometimes buried under old leaves or a shrub, that show where the property line is.

The play space may be sharing the property with other uses, in which case it's important to carefully consider where it will be located. Keep an open mind and pay attention to which spots on the site might really lend themselves to play: a protected niche inside a hedge, a cool overlook, the perfect gnarly tree roots.

Sometimes a community play space is one portion of a larger site at a school, place of worship, or other organization. It may be that since the fence around the old play space has always been in a certain place, no one questions the boundaries. But the very thing that could add tremendous play value to the site might be just outside the current fence. When you begin to rework the boundaries, even a little bit, you may be able to include a climbing hill, a gorgeous shade tree, or even just 3 feet more space that could make a huge difference. I never understand why so many playgrounds seem to place fences in a way that keeps kids away from the most fun stuff!

NATURE iN UNEXPECTED PLACES

Nature may already be there, even if you haven't noticed it. My daughter was a teacher with an after-school writing program in a middle school in southeast Washington, DC, for several years. Based on what she knew about kids, she understood that their restlessness at certain times of the day was a sign that her students needed some time in nature. Outside in their very urban, somewhat neglected schoolyard, she and her students started to look for nature. First, they found mulberries and learned that the dark berries were, lo and behold, safe—and delicious—to eat. After a little trash removal, a concrete-lined creek turned out to have mud, flowing water, and sticks. These ingredients provided the raw materials for imagination and adventure, experiments in lifting, hauling, sculpting, and creating. Many of these almost-teens had never had experiences in nature, and when they took the time to notice what was right outside their door, they were captivated. They marveled at their own resourcefulness and newfound competence as they snacked on berries, wild onions, and honeysuckle nectar, musing, "We could survive out here!" The nature those kids needed was there, it was just a matter of noticing it, and giving them unstructured time to explore.

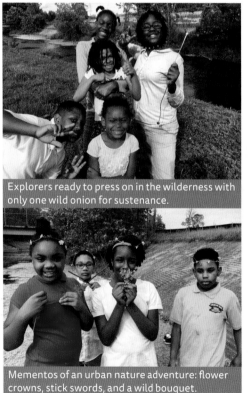

Explorers ready to press on in the wilderness with only one wild onion for sustenance.

Mementos of an urban nature adventure: flower crowns, stick swords, and a wild bouquet.

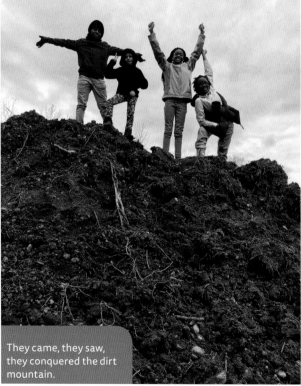

They came, they saw, they conquered the dirt mountain.

Creating a base plan

The next step is to draw a base plan. This is a sheet that shows what is on the site before the new design is created, and it is used as a foundation for the design. The base plan will be incredibly useful, so the more complicated your site and project are, the more important it is to make your base plan as accurate as possible. If your site is very flat and simple, you may only need the length and width of the space. In a site with complex topography, the best thing may be to have a professional surveyor do the measuring for you. They will have laser measuring devices that will guarantee an accurate picture of your space. If you can't use a surveyor, you can get an idea of grade changes by measuring the height of a flight of steps or counting down the bricks on a wall next to the slope.

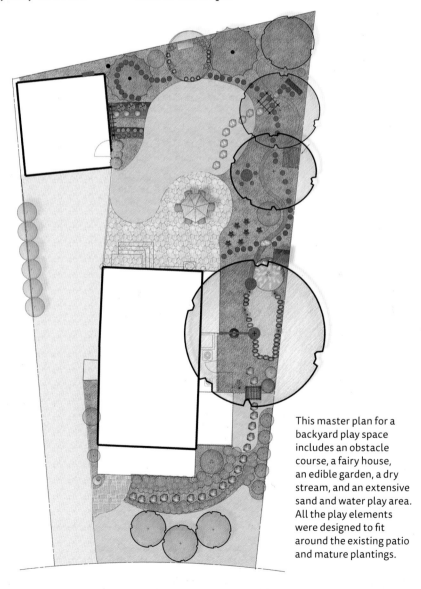

This master plan for a backyard play space includes an obstacle course, a fairy house, an edible garden, a dry stream, and an extensive sand and water play area. All the play elements were designed to fit around the existing patio and mature plantings.

A good way to figure out where something like a tree in the middle of a lawn is located is to create a grid by running straight, parallel lines some set distance apart, say 10 feet. I usually start the grid by measuring some fixed element such as a building or a road. I then locate the fixed features, like trees, on that grid, and transfer it to graph paper. It may help to measure once and then measure again from a different direction. Having a few tape measures is helpful in accurately locating things. Young children love to hold one end of the tape; older ones can be in charge of measuring some portion of the space. It's a great math activity.

Here are the steps to follow:
1. Start with a clipboard and a copy of the plat or site plan. Sketch in things that are in the space but don't show on the plat. If the plat or site plan is not available, sketch the space on a piece of paper. Include everything that will stay in the space, such as sheds, trees, fences, walkways, and existing buildings.* Show the property lines or other edges of the space. Using pens of several colors will help make your notes more readable later—for instance, sketch in blue, add measurements in red, draw in plants with green, make notes in purple.
2. Note sunny spots, shady spots, views you might want to highlight or screen, and places where water flows or collects.
3. Measure and note measurements on your sketch with dimension lines, so you'll remember later where you measured from and to.
4. To get curved edges like walks or beds, measure at fixed intervals off a straight line (such as a fence or building).

5. Redraw the whole thing to scale on graph paper.

*You may leave what you know isn't staying in the space off of your base plan, or you may need to show it if you're not doing the construction work, so that whoever is doing that work will know what to remove.

Someone will have to make decisions about what stays and what goes. Sometimes that's a hard question when people are attached to things. There may need to be conversation and negotiation. There could be history that is important to know, so you can make an informed decision about whether it's possible to repurpose something with sentimental value in the new space. For one family I worked with, the goal was to create a landscape that would be inviting both for visiting grandchildren and as a gathering place for adults. A patio was made of square pavers set in a lush green lawn, but in one corner of the patio, I snuck in the old, battered rubber home plate that reminded the grandfather of his childhood games and honored his beloved lost brother. It was meaningful for him, and it opened the door to stories for his grandchildren.

Reusing and recycling

For whatever can't remain where it is, consider repurposing or recycling. Of course, we want to save trees whenever we can. An arborist can help you to decide if a tree or parts of it are damaged or diseased or for some other reason dangerous. If so, the tree may need to come down. Sometimes it's a little easier to take down a tree if you know that the parts can be repurposed for play. See the chapters titled "Challenging Bodies" and "Inviting Nature" for more on how to use tree parts such as logs, stumps, branches, and snags (the still-standing parts of a dead tree) in play.

Reusing anything that has to be removed is the sustainable approach. Concrete walks, pads, and driveways can be cut up into squares, which are called "urbanite." Urbanite can be stacked to make walls or the foundation of cob structures (see sidebar later in this chapter). If old concrete can't be reused on the site, it can be recycled, to be ground up and used as aggregate in new concrete. Stone and brick can often be reused, but removing old mortar takes time. This may not matter if you are doing the work, but if you're paying a contractor, the extra labor will add to the cost of reuse. Asphalt should always be recycled. Old play equipment can sometimes be taken apart and the components reused: an old slide set into a hillside or ladders repurposed in a new treehouse. If you can't reuse something in your space, letting go of pieces with sentimental value is sometimes easier if they're donated to someone who will appreciate them. Play equipment can be donated; metal can be recycled. There are toxicity risks in using tires, whole or shredded, in any way that children will come in direct contact with the rubber. Dispose of them responsibly. Most municipalities do not allow them in landfills, and have special procedures for tire disposal.

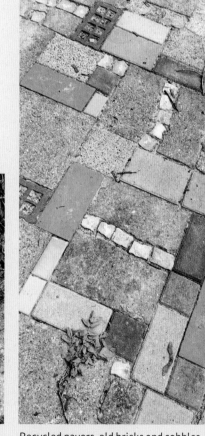

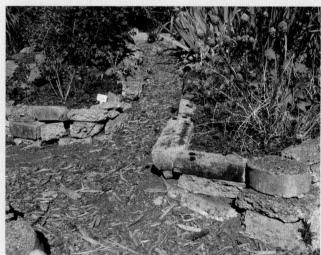

Recycled concrete cut into rough squares can be stacked into garden walls.

Recycled pavers, old bricks and cobbles, are combined in a colorful path.

Deciding what you want

As you get a handle on your existing space and what stays or goes, you will simultaneously be thinking about what you want to do with the space. Don't be afraid to start off dreaming big! As you refine your design, some ideas will be eliminated, but better not to rein yourself in at the beginning.

As a designer in the projects I work on, I'm steering the ship when it comes to creating the design, but I don't do it alone. I don't advise you to go solo, either. Everyone who will use the space needs to be included in the process. Families can browse this book together, then make lists and drawings as a group, or individuals can sketch their own vision and then come together with others to share and combine ideas.

Spend time with your children brainstorming, listing, writing about ideas, drawing your vision, and building models with sand, soil, sticks, leaves, and clay in a tray or a box, or on the ground.

If the space is already being used by children, it is always useful to watch them playing. While they're outside, ask kids to tell you and show you what they like and what's not working in their current play space.

You can also take field trips together to see other natural play spaces, then discuss what inspired them or you (or didn't), and what might be included in your space. Getting everyone involved and feeling ownership in the outcome is an important way to ensure success. Don't forget to talk to neighbors. One early conversation between neighbors can be the difference between complaints to city inspectors and an offer to donate wood for den building.

Mediating ideas

Sometimes in the euphoria of brainstorming, people get attached to ideas that don't seem possible, or visions collide. When that happens, treat every idea with respect, and try hard to find ways to accommodate the spirit of what each person wants. For example, if climbing emerges as an important part of play, but stakeholders are dead set on specific, yet incompatible, climbing elements, try steering the conversation away from individual preferences and toward the many types of climbing experiences possible. One

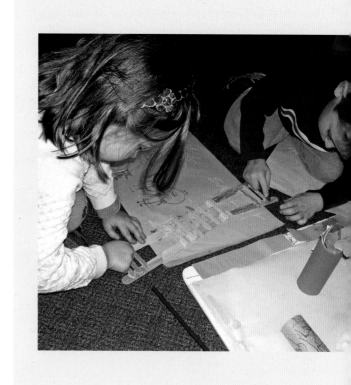

might emerge that suits everyone. Never make promises you can't keep—children remember!

Afterward, pull all the ideas together, and create a written list of elements and design considerations. Check to be sure everyone agrees that the document captures all the ideas in words, and when the list is complete to everyone's satisfaction, it's time to begin drawing the design. After field trips, looking at photos, and talking together, children can write and draw their ideas for the play space.

Building models with blocks, art supplies, or natural materials helps kids explore and communicate their ideas in three dimensions.

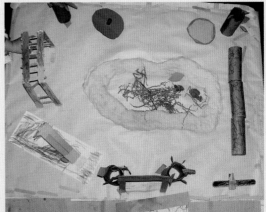

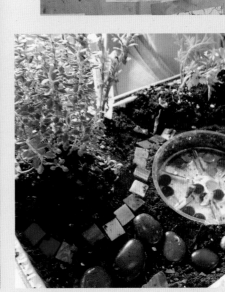

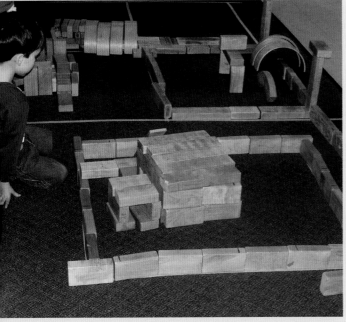

HOW TO RUN A DESIGN CHARETTE

Whether you're trying to create a natural play space for your backyard or your community, consider a design charette—a participatory workshop that brings together everyone who cares about the space and the process to change it. Include members of your family, including children (and teens who may not play in the space, but may use it after hours), and neighbors of all ages. If appropriate, also invite local elected officials, parks staff, teachers, parents, administrators, licensing staff (if it's a childcare facility), property managers and landlords of multifamily buildings, members of the congregation if it's a faith-based site, potential funders—anyone who might have an interest in the project or might provide help in bringing it to fruition. If it's a community space, facilities and maintenance staff are key. There are too many sad stories about gardens that were planted and ponds that were dug without consulting facilities people, then staff came along in their regular duties and mowed under, or filled in, or tore out the elements that had been created. An inclusive process is essential!

In the charette, it is important to start by educating each other. Share this book, including the information about why kids need nature, and ideas about what the space could offer. Break into small groups and brainstorm together. Each group can draw on a base plan and start to play with what could go where. Reconvene and compare ideas.

This kind of event brings people together and offers them a stake in the space. Down the road—when you're fundraising, or looking for workday volunteers, or you need ongoing help to care for the space—that sense of ownership will reap rewards.

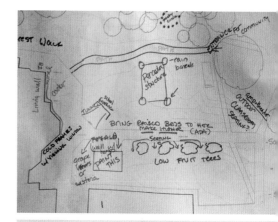

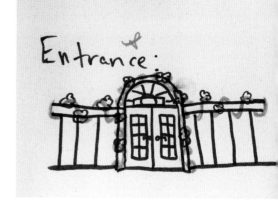

During the design phase, bring together all stakeholders—whether it is those in your family or your community. The best ideas come when everyone is at the table together, brainstorming, writing, drawing, and sharing possibilities.

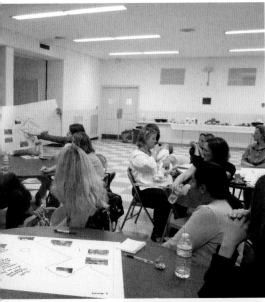

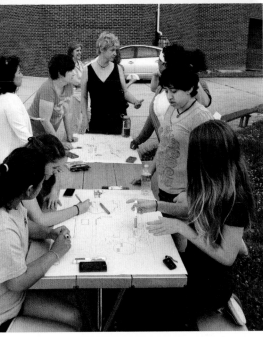

Create your design

The process of creating a design that will work in the space and for the people who'll use it is a bit of a dance, a back and forth, an iterative process, between what the site offers and needs, the resources that are available to you, and what people want. Being aware of this allows you to incorporate recycled elements, donated objects, and easily available materials into your design. At the same time, don't be held hostage to using something that just doesn't fit.

Think about maintaining the space, and what will be required. Don't take on more than you, your family, or your community can realistically handle. Keep playing with the design, sharing it with others, stepping away and looking at it with fresh eyes, and you'll keep getting closer until a solution clicks into place.

There are a couple of ways to approach implementation of your design, and each has advantages. One direction is to create a master plan, thinking through the entire space, considering the overall vision. This can help avoid unanticipated consequences or hurdles down the road. A master plan can be built all at once, but it can also be phased in over time, as the energy and funds become available. Another approach is to start with one project in one corner of the space and design it, build it, play with it, learn from it, and add more later. Either approach can work.

No matter the scale of your design, a good first step to getting it on paper is to use a technique that designers call bubble diagrams. Begin by sketching amorphous shapes to show the relative size and adjacency of the elements you want to include in the space. Think about the elements on your list, and what thing makes sense located near a particular something else. Think about how people currently move through the space (sometimes described as "paths of desire") and how they will move through the future space, and then sketch in pathways early in the process. The layout of pathways will define islands in between and those can become outdoor rooms. Your rough sketches will keep getting revised and refined, details will be added and materials determined, and the plan will become more and more precise. Eventually you will have a beautiful, colorful, scale drawing of the space. It can hang on the wall and serve as an inspiration and a roadmap forward. If this is a community project, your drawing can communicate the plan to the wider community and help in fundraising.

If your project is large or complicated, or if you just feel somewhat unclear or overwhelmed, you may want to call in a professional designer. This person can help translate the ideas and guidelines in this book into a plan that will work in your yard or community. A designer can help you to decide on materials, create a planting plan, and figure out how things should be constructed. Designers can also help in navigating the complexities of permitting and hiring a contractor, and can oversee construction to ensure it's happening according to plan.

Safety and risk

As discussed throughout this book, it is important to pay attention to safety during construction and in the space you create. There are national safety standards for manufactured play equipment and much of the logic behind those guidelines can be applied to natural play spaces. Become familiar with these guidelines. Think about the area around the element—a fallen tree or a boulder, for example, and the surfacing you plan to use. A great deal of testing and research has been done to determine fall heights and the potential of injuries. Grass on soil does not create an adequate safety surface. Sand or a thick layer of mulch or wood chips is safer. Think about areas of entrapment, where children could get parts of their bodies stuck. Watch out for protrusions that could poke. Check out playground-safety.org/standards/cpsc for specific guidelines.

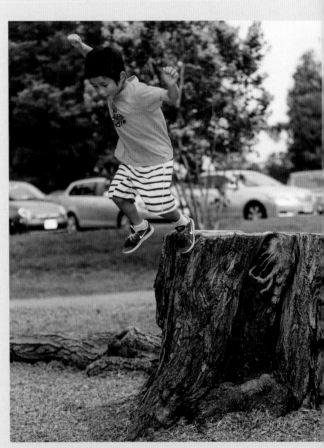

Wood chip surfacing provides a natural look and offers a soft landing.

There are some who contend that when safety guidelines were created, not enough attention was given to children's wisdom and ability to make good choices. You will want to balance the potential for beneficial risk-taking with the need to reduce chances of serious injury. When a child has the opportunity to know their own abilities and to consider what they feel comfortable doing, we give them an opportunity to understand themselves and to learn valuable decision-making skills. The position of the International School Grounds Alliance (internationalschoolgrounds.org/risk/), referenced earlier and backed by research from around the globe, states, "Since the world is full of risks, children need to learn how to recognize and respond to them in order to protect themselves and to develop their own risk-assessment capabilities." More on risk can be found in the "Challenging Bodies" chapter.

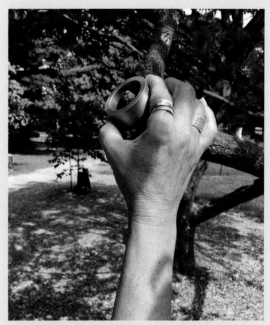

Using a protrusion gauge, the CPSI checks a stub that needs to be trimmed off this branch so as not to injure a child. Pay attention to safety guidelines, and balance reasonable care with giving kids the opportunity to learn to make good choices.

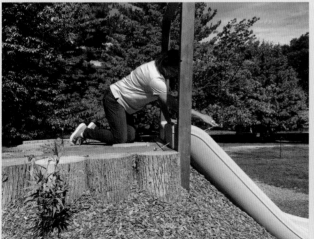 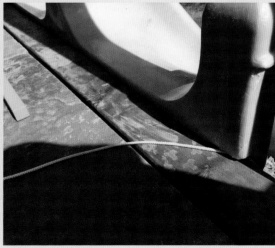

The goal is to make spaces safe enough to prevent frequent or serious injuries. A certified playground safety inspector (CPSI) finds that the top of this slide needs some caulk to prevent hood strings from getting caught.

FUNDING YOUR PLAY SPACE

A project becomes very real when costs are considered. As the design is coming together, it's helpful to think about the funds and resources you have available (or think you can come up with), and to design accordingly. It may be worthwhile to do some early research into the costs of materials and make design decisions based on what works *and* what you can afford. Show the plans to a contractor if you plan on using one, and get input into the costs of potential materials and the labor required for different building techniques. Keep those costs in mind as you design. Found objects, recycling, and DIY aspects of construction are all ways to make the transformation affordable on even the most modest budget.

Sometimes, especially if you're using contractors who charge for each hour of their time, you'll find that recycled materials are not less expensive because of the time involved in procuring or preparing them. This may come as disappointing news, but chipping old mortar off bricks takes time and may make recycled pavers, though beautiful, a more expensive option. It's important to go into this with eyes wide open.

On the other hand, one person's yard discards can be someone else's treasured loose parts. The more word spreads about nature play, the more people will recognize the value of readily available natural materials for such spaces. Post on your neighborhood listserv and offer to pick up materials if someone is taking a tree down,

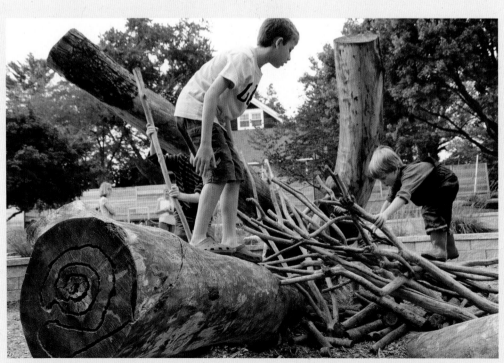

Downed trees and tree parts can be affordable play space additions, if you can source them from an arborist or tree service.

pruning their curly willow, or thinning bamboo. If you're the one doing the cutting, let your neighbors know it will be there for the taking. As mentioned previously, your local tree company or arborist may become your best friend. Trees are always coming down, and while sometimes that wood is sold as lumber or firewood, it often must be hauled to a disposal site. If a tree company knows you're in the market for specific types of wood and they are taking down trees of that variety nearby, they may be quite happy to drop it off.

As you go forward, you'll come upon some choices. If we pay to have this built it will cost this much in dollars, and if we build it ourselves it will take this much time. If we reuse this material we will save this amount, and if we buy it new, it will cost this much. If we bundle all these tasks together the overall cost (and disruption) will be less, and if we phase it in over time we will have a chance to save up and learn from each step. Compile as much information as possible, then make the best decisions you can to balance and allocate the available time, expertise, energy, and funding you have.

For neighborhood play spaces, you will want to consider each person's resources and abilities, and what they can contribute. Some people can provide skilled or unskilled labor, others can offer funds, and yet others can raise funds.

If you decide to go out into the community to raise funds, you will need visuals—photos, along with your drawings—that inspire and communicate your goals in a compelling way. Use this book if certain images or ideas found here convey elements you want to incorporate. You can approach the community in a variety of ways. A cost can be assigned to each element in the space

and families, grandparents, and neighbors can "buy a log" and have their name on a sign in the space. You can approach businesses and foundations in your community for funding, or hold events like yard sales, concerts, spelling bees, and running races to raise funds. There can be workdays where big groups come together to do the work of creating the space: building, digging, moving, planting, and painting. You'll want to provide food and childcare for those types of work parties. Or individuals or teams can take on a task and complete it at their own pace within a schedule.

BUILDING YOUR PLAY SPACE

However you decide to create your play area, there is a rough but logical sequence to landscape construction that you should try to follow for every project, large and small.

The first step is to protect the trees and soil that are staying. This may mean putting fencing around trees so that heavy tools and materials won't be piled on their roots. It may mean placing silt fencing so that if it rains after you've just dug a big hole, mud won't run off into storm drains. Depending on where you live, your local jurisdiction may have rules to protect trees and your watershed during construction. Find out what those rules are and abide by them.

When you start construction, the goal is to do the most disruptive things first. That means installing anything underground like pipes or drains or wiring, and getting any digging or grading done at the beginning. The next step is to install anything that will require heavy equipment, such as boulders, large tree parts, and hardscaping. After that, tackle the elements that

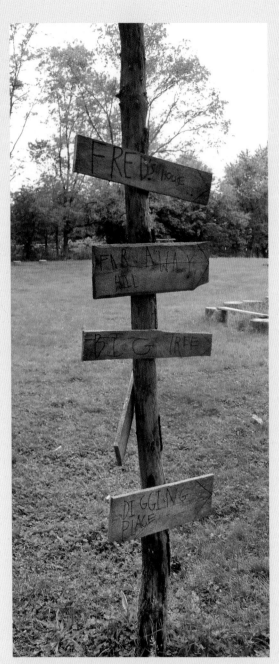

Naming important landmarks helps create a sense of place. Child-made signs are a chance to practice reading and writing and bring literacy outside.

require carpentry, such as fences and sheds and pergolas. Pour concrete walks and lay paving after the chance of driving over it with construction machines is past. Finally, prepare the beds and add plants, from large to small: trees first, then shrubs, then grasses and perennials, and finally lawn or sod. This sequence applies even if you're only transforming one corner of a yard. The goal is always to avoid tearing up something that is already in place, so don't install anything without first making sure that the previous steps are complete in that portion of the space.

Whether it is to save money or because you're bursting with creative energy, there are huge benefits to creating at least a little bit of your space yourself *and* getting your kids involved. The experience is important, fun, and will save money. It will give you and your child that sense of pride and ownership that comes from doing it with your own hands.

Hiring experts

At any point in the process, if you find your vision exceeds your abilities, don't be afraid to bring in a landscape professional. It may make perfect sense for you to hire a skilled designer to create a plan that you later build yourself, or you may want a contractor to build what you've designed—or both. There may also be rules from insurers or communities that define what can and cannot be done by volunteers or nonprofessionals.

Whatever your process, just watching your play space get built can create a tremendous sense of excitement. It is a special opportunity for children to see how it's done and to see the materials and tools that are used.

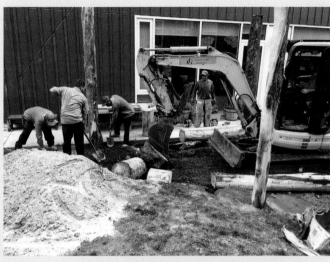

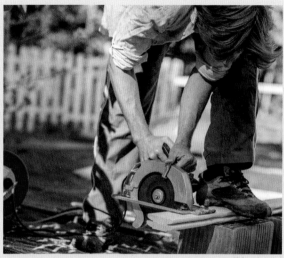

Digging a sandpit and installing edging happens quickly with a team of professionals and their equipment.

You may have skills that make building a nature play space on your own a smart (and cost-effective) decision.

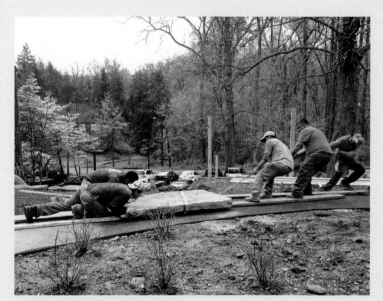

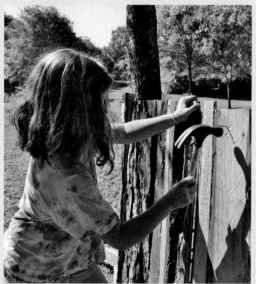

It may be wise to hire a crew to move large stones or boulders, especially up a slope.

If you decide to do all or a portion of the work yourself, there will be jobs for all ages.

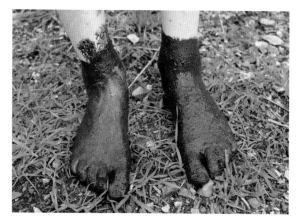

A fun and important aspect of the cob construction process.

THE PLAY SPACE THAT MUDDY FEET BUILT

A playground improvement I worked on for Clarendon Child Care Center (CCCC) was not a backyard home project, but there are valuable takeaways from it that apply to natural play space construction anywhere.

The story begins with the wish for a new playhouse. The new director of CCCC approached me because their beloved playhouse had been loved to death and needed to be replaced. Her recently retired predecessor had asked that her retirement gift be improvements to their playground. There were a number of issues that needed to be addressed beyond the original playhouse, and the final renovation included many natural play elements, but the anchors of the project would be three structures: two playhouses and a shunnel (shed/tunnel). Having more than one playhouse would encourage conversation and social interaction among the children who would use them.

As with many projects (both home and community based), the undertaking was defined not just by the space, but by those involved and their skills or connections. We had a contact at the county office, through the CCCC board president, who supported sustainability and green building. We also knew a wonderful man in the area who had recently retired. He had been studying and experimenting with cob construction and straw-bale building and was passionate about sharing these techniques. The decision was made to partner with the county, who would offer a series of classes in natural building techniques in the play space, led by the retiree. The play structures

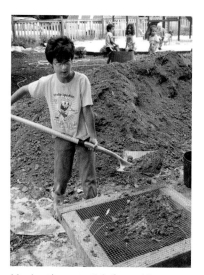

Moving the materials for making cob—soil, sand, straw, and water—is good work for kids' proprioceptive development. The traditional way to mix ingredients is with bare feet.

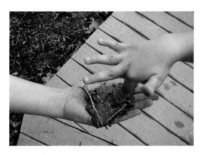

Just right!

would then be built by volunteers and class members, the play-houses from cob and the shunnel out of straw bales covered in a natural lime plaster. The shunnel would have a living roof, and the playhouse roofs would be wood shake.

Cob construction is a type of natural building that uses clayey soil, sand, and straw, mixed with water, to build buildings out of wet bricks called "cobs." Cob is a word from the British Islands meaning "loaf," so cobs are blobs of mud about the size of a loaf of bread. These are formed, stacked, and sculpted so that as they dry, the structures are smooth and organic looking. Cob is incredibly durable as long as it has, as cob-bers say, "dry feet and a dry head," which means a good foundation that keeps the cob off the ground and a solid roof with big over-hangs to protect the walls. There

are cob houses in Great Britain that are more than 500 years old.

Straw bale construction uses materials similar to cob, but in a different way. Building on a foun-dation, whole bales are stacked, anchored, and plastered over with natural plaster—either earth plaster (made of clay, sand, water, and shredded paper) or lime (made of a limestone mix that hardens when exposed to air), to seal out moisture. Like cob, straw bale construction needs a roof with a good overhang to help pro-tect it from weather.

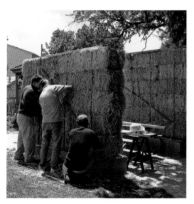

The straw-bale shunnel was made by stacking bales on a cement block foundation poured and cured in advance. Bales were fastened together with strapping.

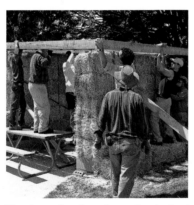

The shunnel roof was framed and raised onto the straw bale walls. Plywood decking, a waterproof layer, and metal edging were installed next. Walls were sealed with a natural lime plaster.

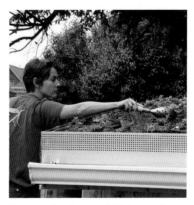

Trays on the shunnnel's living roof were filled with a Rooflite growing medium and planted with hundreds of succulents.

One of the most desirable aspects of natural building with cob and straw bales is that it can be done using no power tools and for very little cost, making it well suited to involving children. Another advantage of cob building is that the traditional way to mix the soil, sand, and straw is with bare feet. Who can resist ooshy-squooshy mud? (Some kids definitely can—and that's okay!)

About one to two feet of wall can be built in one session.

Then it needs to set up for a few days. PVC pipe was embedded in one wall of each house and connected underground, so the finished houses would be connected by a whisper phone. Sound carries through the PVC tube, so kids can talk and be heard between the houses.

Classes and building happened throughout the summer—and what a summer it was! Lots of workdays, lots of mud, and lots of amazing people who gave their time and energy to

help us build. Over many Saturdays, we drew class members as well as different groups to help us build. One day was a workshop for early childhood teachers who were earning training credit. Another group was a reunion of alumni from the childcare center, so a group of fourth-grade boys and their parents gleefully reconnected in the mud. Builders included church members, scout troops, and friends from the local elementary and high school. Passersby would stop

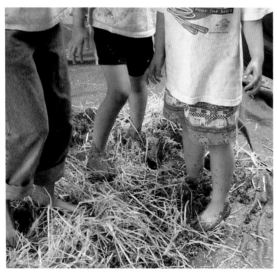

Children delight in mixing soil, sand, straw, and water with their bare feet to create cob for building.

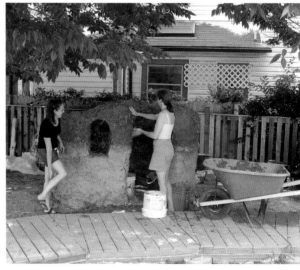

Volunteers bonded over playing in the mud.

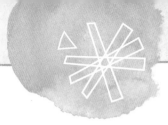

and ask what we were doing, only to soon decide to join us in our muddy fun. Many days were gatherings of the Washington, DC, green-building community, who honed their skills as they visited in the mud. A U.S. State Department envoy returning from Afghanistan came and told us about multi-storied mud structures in Kabul, as we stomped together in the mud. A young consultant who was working to green the Pentagon came to dig his toes in the mud and was eventually employed by the county to work in their energy conservation program. Bonding in mud builds community!

Natural building takes time, though. It was about seven months before everything was completed, certainly a bigger project than anyone imagined at the start. But it was also a powerful experience for everyone involved. We spent countless hours from early April until late in the fall, almost every weekend and Wednesday night, organizing dozens of generous volunteers and participating in work sessions to get those little structures built. A culture of caring was born that summer and thrives to this day at the center. By the arrival of the cold fall that ensued, we had built a wonderful play space—as well as deep friendships of the sort that only come from hours together, toes immersed in mud.

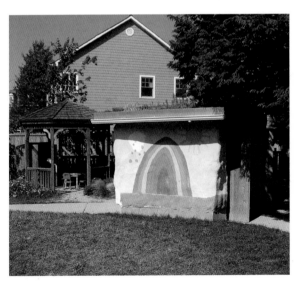

Children worked with an artist to paint a rainbow mural on the finished shunnel.

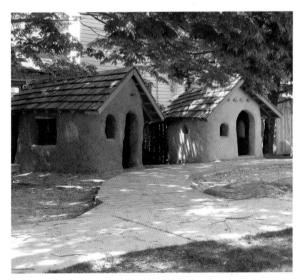

One playhouse was sealed with North Carolina red-clay plaster, the other with white-clay plaster from Alexandria, Virginia. (Foundations have been obscured by sand.)

MAINTENANCE DISGUISED AS FUN

Reducing the spread of invasive plants is something we all can help with—even kids, when the outcome is a fun (though ephemeral) natural play space. This group of children spent a school field day culling invasive plant vines and using the vines to build a couple of pole huts connected by a tunnel. Materials were bamboo poles and cut vines of English ivy and kudzu—all of which are invasive. If someone you know has any of these plants in their yard, they will likely be delighted to let you harvest some!

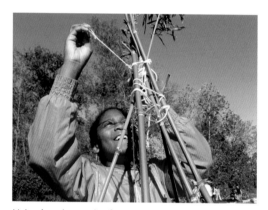

Using bamboo poles from an invasive patch, children constructed two huts, with the tops tied together by string.

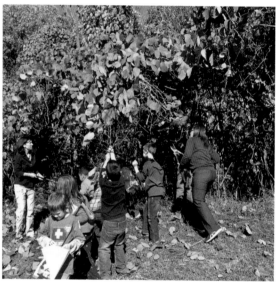

First, vines of English ivy and kudzu were cut and collected.

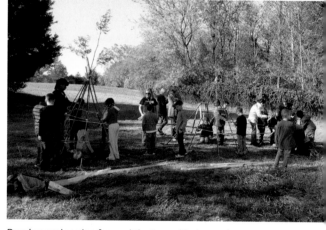

Bamboo poles also framed the tunnel between huts.

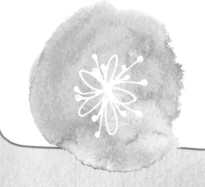

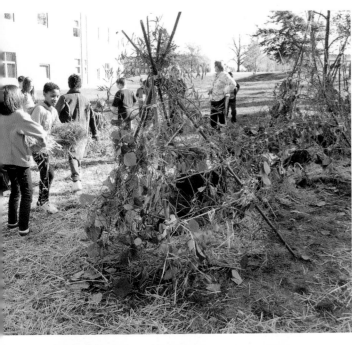

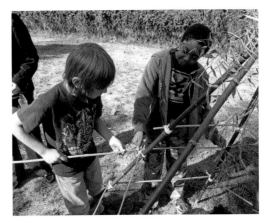

Smaller bamboo support stakes were used as cross pieces to increase the huts' stability.

Cut vines were draped and woven around huts and tunnel frames, creating a sense of enclosure.

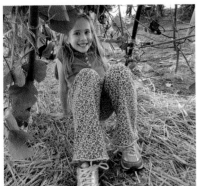

Straw was spread as a soft floor for the huts and tunnel.

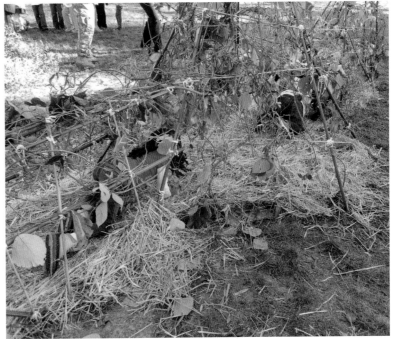

CARING FOR YOUR PLAY SPACE

There is no such thing as a maintenance-free space. No matter what you create, some care will be required. Some of the typical tasks in a natural play space have to do with replacing things that break down or vanish. Decomposition and rotting are natural processes and part of the learning available to children who play in nature. Logs and stumps will decay over time, loose parts will disappear along with sand and mulch. All those things may need to be replenished. Sand and mulch will migrate, so providing brooms and rakes will help children participate in caring for their space. Weeds will need to be pulled; branches may need to be trimmed. Those branches and weeds can be composted, used as play props, or even used as part of a natural tapestry in a weaving project. There are some tasks that need to happen regularly—every day or at least once a week. These include checking the space for hazards like broken glass or nails,

gathering trash, putting things away so they're accessible for play, and maybe raking and sweeping where it's needed. Plants should be watered and weeded.

Consider that the space will always be adjusting to meet the changing needs of children. Maintenance is an opportunity to bring in new elements and respond to kids' ever-changing interests. Best of all, evolution is a sign of success—proof that you have made a great investment in your property, in being ecologically responsible, and in the lives of all who are lucky enough to enjoy the wonders and lessons of your natural play space.

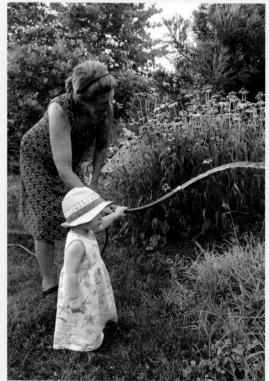

Involving children in caring for living things helps to develop empathy and responsibility.

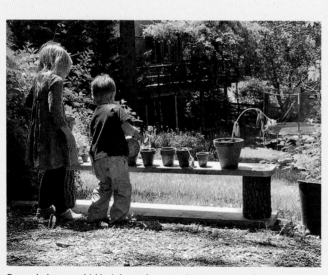

Potted plants at kid height make watering an easy task.

METRIC CONVERSIONS

INCHES	CENTIMETERS
¼	0.6
⅓	0.8
½	1.25
1	2.5
2	5.0
3	7.5
4	10
5	12.5
6	15
7	18
8	20
9	23
10	25

FEET	METERS
¼	0.08
⅓	0.1
½	0.15
1	0.3
2	0.6
3	0.9
4	1.2
5	1.5
6	1.8
7	2.1
8	2.4
9	2.7
10	3.0

TEMPERATURES

°C ? ⁵⁄₉ χ (°F / 32)

°F ? (⁹⁄₅ χ °C) , 32

REFERENCES

INTRODUCTION

Derbyshire, David, "How children lost the right to roam in four generations," *Daily Mail*, June 15, 2007.

Grahn, Patrik, Fredrika Mårtensson, Bodil Lindblad, Paula Nilsson, and Anna Ekman, "Ute pa Dagis," *Stad & Land* 145.

Louv, Richard, *Last Child in the Woods: Saving Our Children from Nature-Deficit Disorder*. Chapel Hill, North Carolina: Algonquin Books, 2005.

Olds, Anita Rui, *The Child Care Design Guide*. New York: McGraw Hill, 2001.

White, Jan, and Helen Woolley, "What Makes a Good Outdoor Environment for Young Children" in *Exploring Outdoor Play in the Early Years*, ed. Trisha Maynard and Jane Waters. Berkshire, England: McGraw-Hill Education, 2014.

AWAKENING SENSES

"Getting Dirty May Lift Your Mood," *University of Bristol News*, April 2, 2007.

Lowry, C.A. et al., "Identification of an immune-responsive mesolimbocortical serotonergic system: Potential role in regulation of emotional behavior," *Neuroscience* 146: 756–772.

Palmer, Brian, "Why Are So Many Kids Getting Myopia? Spending Time Indoors May Impair Children's Vision." *Slate*, October 16, 2013, slate.com/articles/health_and_science/medical_examiner/2013/10/myopia_increasing_indoor_light_may_be_impairing_children_s_vision.html.

Piff, Paul K. et al, "Awe, the Small Self, and Prosocial Behavior," *Journal of Personality and Social Psychology* 108: 883–899.

CHALLENGING BODIES

Akerblom, Dr. Petter, Lecture, International School Grounds Alliance Conference, "Engaging our Grounds," San Francisco, CA, 2011.

Almon, Joan, *Adventure: The Value of Risk in Child's Play*. CreateSpace Independent Publishing Platform, 2013.

Ball, David, Bernard Spiegel, and Tim Gill, *Managing Risk in Play Provision: Implementation Guide*. playengland.org.uk/resource/aging-risk-in-play-provision-implementation-guide/.

Collyer, Cam, Lecture, International School Grounds Alliance Conference, "Engaging our Grounds," San Francisco, CA, 2011.

Hanscom, Angela, *Balanced and Barefoot*. Oakland, California: New Harbinger Publications, 2016.

International School Grounds Alliance. *Risk in Play and Learning: Ubud-Höör Declaration*. internationalschoolgrounds.org/risk/.

Miyazaki, Yoshifumi, *Shinrin-Yoku: The Japanese Art of Forest Bathing*. Portland, Oregon: Timber Press, 2018.

Olds, Anita Rui, from "Cartwheels to Caterpillars: The Child's Need for Motion Outdoors." *Human Ecology Forum* 10: 25.

Rosin, Hanna, "The Overprotected Kid," *The Atlantic*, April 2014.

Sandseter, Ellen Beate Hansen and Leif Edward Ottesen Kennair, "Children's Risky Play from an Evolutionary Perspective: The Anti-Phobic Effects of Thrilling Experiences," *Evolutionary Psychology* 9 (2): 257–284.

Spiegal, Dr. Bernard, Lecture, International School Grounds Alliance Conference, "Engaging our Grounds," San Francisco, CA, 2011.

Striniste, Nancy and Robin Moore, "Early Childhood Outdoors: A Literature Review Related to the Design of Childcare Environments." *Children's Environments Quarterly* 6 (4): 25–31.

"Study: Natural Playgrounds More Beneficial to Children, Inspire More Play." *The University of Tennessee Knoxville News*, October 11, 2012.

U.S. Consumer Product Safety Commission, *Outdoor Home Playground Safety Handbook*. cpsc.gov/s3fs-public/324.pdf.

U.S. Consumer Product Safety Commission, *Public Playground Safety Handbook*. cpsc.gov/s3fs-public/325.pdf.

INVITING NATURE

Kuo, Frances E. and Andrea F. Taylor "A potential natural treatment for attention-deficit/hyperactivity disorder: Evidence from a national study." *American Journal of Public Health* 94 (9): 1580–1586.

Louv, Richard, *Last Child in the Woods: Saving Our Children from Nature-Deficit Disorder*. Chapel Hill, North Carolina: Algonquin Books, 2005.

Smith, Laura, "Rx: 50 mg Nature, Ad Lib: Doctors are prescribing a walk in the park." *Slate*, July 25, 2014, slate.com/articles/health_and_science/medical_examiner/2014/07/doctors_prescribing_outdoors_time_nature_is_good_for_you.html.

Tallamy, Douglas, *Bringing Nature Home: How Native Plants Sustain Wildlife in Our Gardens*. Portland, Oregon: Timber Press, 2007.

Taylor, Andrea F., Frances E. Kuo, and William C. Sullivan, "Coping with ADD: The Surprising Connection to Green Play Settings." *Environment and Behavior* 33 (1): 54–77.

Ulrich, R.S., "View through a window may influence recovery from surgery." Science 224 (4647): 420–421.

RESOURCES

BOOKS

Danks, Sharon Gamson. 2010. *Asphalt to Ecosystems: Design Ideas for Schoolyard Transformation*. Oakland, California: New Village Press.

Dannenmaier, Molly. 1998. *A Child's Garden: Enchanting Outdoor Spaces for Children and Parents*. New York: Simon & Schuster Editions.

Denzer, Kiko. 2005. *Dig Your Hands in the Dirt! A manual for making art out of earth*. Philomath, OR: Hand Print Press.

Denzer, Kiko and Hannah Field. 2007. *Build Your Own Earth Oven: A Low-Cost Wood-Fired Mud Oven, Simple Sourdough Bread, Perfect Loaves*. Philomath, Oregon: Hand Print Press.

Dunnett, Nigel, Dusty Gedge, John Little, and Edmund Snodgrass. 2011. *Small Green Roofs* Portland, Oregon: Timber Press.

Evans, Ianto, Michael G. Smith, and Linda Smiley. 2002. *The Hand Sculpted House: A Practical and Philosophical Guide to Building a Cob Cottage*. White River Junction, Vermont: Chealsea Green Publishing Company.

Greenman, Jim. 2005. *Caring Spaces, Learning Places: Children's Environments That Work*. Redmond, Washington: Exchange Press.

Guinness, Bunny. 2008. *Family Gardens: How to Create Magical Outdoor Spaces for All Ages*. Cincinnati, Ohio: David & Charles.

Kaplan, Rachel and Steven Kaplan. 1980. *The Experience of Nature: A Psychological Perspective*. Cambridge, UK: Cambridge University Press.

Keeler, Rusty. 2008. *Natural Playscapes*. Redmond, Washington: Exchange Press.

Lovejoy, Sharon. 1991. *Sunflower Houses: A Book for Children and Their Grown-Ups*. New York: Workman Publishing.

Moore, Robin. 2014. *Nature Play and Learning Places. Creating and managing places where children engage with nature*. Raleigh, North Carolina: Natural Learning Initiative; Reston, Virginia: National Wildlife Federation.

Moore, Robin and Herb H. Wong. 1997. *Natural Learning: The Life History of an Environmental Schoolyard*. Berkeley, California: MIG Communications.

Rivkin, Mary S. 1995. *The Great Outdoors: Restoring Children's Right to Play Outside*. Washington, DC: National Association for the Education of Young Children.

Sobel, David. 1996. *Beyond Ecophobia*. Great Barrington, Massachusetts: The Orion Society.

Sullivan, Virginia and Wendy Banning. 2011. *Lens on Outdoor Learning*. St. Paul, Minnesota: Red Leaf Press.

White, Jan. 2012. *Making a Mud Kitchen*. Sheffield, England: Muddy Faces Ltd.

White, Jan. 2014. *Playing and Learning Outdoors*. New York: Routledge.

DESIGN

Sigi Koko, architect and natural building expert, Down to Earth Design. buildnaturally.com.

GARDEN SIGNS AND PLANT LABELS

SmartGardenSigns.org

INVASIVE PLANTS BY REGION

Theinvasiveplantatlas.org

NATIVE BEES AND PROVIDING HABITAT FOR THEM

The Xerces Society. xerces.org

NURSERIES AND PLANT SOURCES

Vermont Willow Nursery. willowsvermont.com. Lists more than 20 North American native willow varieties on the website and sells kits for making a variety of willow structures including a tunnel, dome, and fedge (fence + hedge).

Bluestem Nursery. bluestem.ca. Sells willows.

EarthPlay. earthplay.net. Sells willow whips in three different varieties.

Lakeshore Willows. lakeshorewillows.com. Sells kits for playhouses and tunnels, plus many varieties of willow whips.

ORGANIZATIONS

Cornell Lab of Ornithology. birds.cornell.edu. Educational and research resources on birds. Webcams trained on active nests.

National Wildlife Federation. nwf.org. A wealth of information on supporting wildlife, including how to certify your backyard or schoolyard.

The National Audubon Society. audubon.org. Information on birds, how to make your backyard bird-friendly, and citizen science for your family, including the Christmas bird count.

Eastern Regional Association of Forest and Nature Schools. ERAFANS.org.

North American Alliance for Environmental Education. NAAEE.org. Includes the Natural Start Alliance, which supports early childhood environmental education.

Children and Nature Network. childrenandnature.org. Founded by Richard Louv. Resource for everything related to children and nature; especially valuable for their compilation of research.

OUTDOOR MUSICAL INSTRUMENTS

earthplay.net

Weenotes: from freenotesharmonypark.com

soundplay.com

PLANT TOXICITY

North Carolina State University. https://plants.ces.ncsu.edu/plants/category/poisonous-plants/

TREE PARTS

local parks departments, urban foresters, arborists

TWIG PLAYHOUSES, EASELS AND LOOMS, CARVED ANIMALS, HILLSIDE SLIDES

The EarlySpace Shop. earlyspace.com

WEAVING

The Earthloom Foundation. earthloom.org. Curriculum information on weaving plus building plans for your own earth loom.

ACKNOWLEDGMENTS

I am very grateful to so many wise and generous people. I have tried to remember everyone, but inevitably I won't and for any omissions I apologize in advance.

Thanks to Joanne Shoemaker and the late Joan Bergstrom, my teachers at Wheelock College, whose images of Scandinavian childcare in the late '70s first revealed to me that children's spaces could be beautiful; Anita Olds, lost to us too soon, whose Child Care Design classes and institute at Tufts and Harvard Graduate School of Design were life changing. I'm grateful to Sue Reed, Carrie Pekor, and all the teachers, children, and parents I worked with at WCCC, Soldiers Field Park Children's Center, Beginnings, Children's Greenhouse, and Newtowne School; to Robin Moore, teacher, mentor, colleague, and friend whose support and encouragement were pivotal and whose writing and work at NCSU and around the world was an endless resource and inspiration; and to the founders of Playspace at City Market in Raleigh and the administrators at RDU who initiated the PlayPort project there.

I'm indebted to Art Scherer and his work at Go Out and Play, and all the contractors (especially Jeff Potter of J&G Landscaping and Tom Hunt of GEL) who've taken a chance to build my designs; to Family Preschool, Duke School, McDougle School, Carolina Friends School, Christine Alvarado and East Coast Migrant Head Start, Seawell and Lincoln Head Start programs, Clarendon Child Care Center, Silver Spring Day School, Montessori School of Northern Virginia, Drew Model School, Mundo Verde and Creative Minds International Public Charter Schools, Bender JCC, the City of Gaithersburg, Lowell School, Fort Belvoir Elementary, Campbell Elementary School, Key Elementary School, Tuckahoe Elementary School, and Westlawn Elementary School, and all the passionate teachers, parents, administrators, and others at all the homes, schools, and childcare programs I've had the privilege to work with.

Thanks to Janet McGinnis, who led the Outdoor Learning Environments Project that launched years of good work in North Carolina and Nancy Easterling of the North Carolina Botanical Garden for sharing a wealth of plant lore; Janet Turchi, the model for my ideal client and still a dear friend; and Giles Blunden, an excellent collaborator who also led my family to our beloved cohousing community; Margaret and David and all of the wonderful adults and children at Arcadia, where childhood was truly muddy and magical; all of our parenting friends

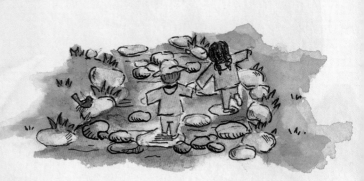

over the years, especially the Parkinsons, with whom we shared many outdoor adventures; to our wonderful neighbors on 19th Street; Beth Reese and the whole gang at Taproot Farm; all my colleagues and friends at NoVA Outside, including Elenor Hodges, Elaine Tholen, Melanie Meren, Peggy Ashbrook, Sissy Walker, and especially Sandra Redmore (and Joan Kelsh) of CCCC.

Appreciation to the first partners at EarlySpace: Deanne Jackson, Diane Gillis, Patti Cruickshank-Schott; to Cheryl Corson, Sandi Olek, and the other members of the Maryland Natural Play space Working Group; the short-lived but brilliant Seneca Creek Collaborative, the design team who took me to the next level along with Chris Sonne, the kindest, most out-of-the-box thinking engineer ever, and Jeff Potter, Charles Kemper, Zech Zorner, and the rest of the talented and dedicated J&G Landscaping team, who, with skill and patience, built many of the spaces in this book. Thanks to my pioneering grad students at Antioch's Nature-Based Early Childhood Education program; my guides in Berlin and Uppsala, especially Manfred Dietzen of Grun Macht Schule, Petter Akerblom of Movium, and Mark Harris and Lotta Frenander. Sissy Walker, Peggy Ashbrook, Carolyn Connell, Jim Chung, and Jesse Chung offered their thoughtful comments on this manuscript, and Betsy Washington, my extraordinary plants teacher at GWU, provided helpful additions to the plant lists. Sigi Koko of Build Naturally and Ed Raduazzo taught me all I know about the magic of natural building. Thank you to all my teachers at GWU, including most especially Lauren Wheeler, and to Sylvan Kaufman, who invited

me to write for the Conservation Landscape Alliance, and Carleen Madigan, who read what I wrote and connected me with the wonderful people at Timber Press.

I especially thank Stacee Lawrence, Julie Talbot, Mary Winkelman Velgos, and the team at Timber, who understood what I wanted to do and promised that this would be a beautiful book. The visionary photographers Lani Harmon, Mark Harris, Brita Monaco, and Amy McGuire captured, with such astute eyes, the spaces I designed and the children who played in them.

Gratitude to Rusty Keeler for his generosity, and thanks to the kids and teachers at Fort Belvoir for inviting me to play. The list of plants for a living roof was assembled with help from Emory Knoll Farms—thank you! Appreciation to Sharon Danks for her inspiration, and to Earth-Loom Foundation. Thanks to the parents who shared photos of their beautiful children: Adam and Laurie, Stephanie, Andrea, Melanie, Jennifer, Jenn, Kate, Emma and Kaia and to all the parents who allowed photos of their children to be included in this book. I cannot adequately thank Rebecca Fox Stoddard and Andrew Stoddard for their incredible generosity in sharing photographs of the wonderful work they do in their beautiful home-based school. Jen Ren started as a student intern and soon revealed herself to be not only organized, efficient, and fun to work with, but also an incredibly talented artist. Her whimsical watercolors brighten this book. Thanks to Christine Kane, who introduced me to the world of upleveling; to Amira Alvarez, duck wrangler extraordinaire, whose teaching inspires me in business and in life; and to Carolyn, Sue, and the other heroic women of the M-7 who helped me to believe that I could do this!

It all began with my own family: my mother and aunts, who sent me outdoors "till the street-lights come on"; my older sister and brother and my sweet stepsisters; my cousins and childhood friends who shared adventures like digging the day lily bulbs in the lilac grove in our yard on Franklin Street. I had magical summers with my cousins in Montague at Gramma's school house: catching minnows in the brook, eating wild blue-berries, picking bouquets of wildflowers, swim-ming in Vi's pond. I treasure my Chung extended family and all of my dear nieces and nephews who played outside with joy in the woods and on the beaches.

Sincere appreciation to my own children most of all. Abbey's patience and focus on tiny salamanders and sculpting with North Caro-lina red clay led to lyrical stories that reveal how much she noticed, soaked up, and became who she is today through her time outside, especially at Arcadia. It was sometimes a challenge to get little boy Jesse away from those enticing screens, but he turned out to be the most passionate and adventurous one of all in his love of wild places. I am pretty sure we owe some part of it to his sum-mers at Burgundy Center for Wildlife Studies, the perfect blend of science, spirit, and silliness, with a very wise leader, Vini Schoene.

And finally, thanks to Jim, my husband and my best friend. His support allowed me to pur-sue this passion for designing spaces for chil-dren through the early years before it became a real job. He was always there to fix my com-puter, order the takeout, and most of all, to keep me laughing through the frustrating times. We shared a commitment to raising our children to love the outdoors—from building backyard swings, sandboxes, and zip lines, to tromping through Shenandoah and the Everglades. We got them outside and it mattered.

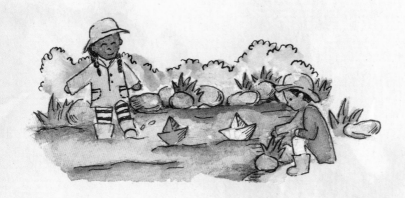

CREDITS

PHOTO, ILLUSTRATION, LOCATION, AND DESIGN CREDITS

PHOTOGRAPHERS

All photographs by the author except the following:

Alamy/Paul Mogford, page 75

Abbey Otis Chung, pages 86 upper right, 216 all

James C. Chung, pages 10, 12 left, 36 center left, 41 top, 55 bottom right, 102 top right, 106 bottom right, 110 bottom right, 125 bottom right, 144 bottom, 152 upper left, 180 top left, 196 bottom left

City of Gaithersburg, Amy McGuire, pages 2, 17, 63 upper cluster: top left and right, lower cluster: upper left; 69 upper right, bottom center, bottom right; 84 center left and right, 88 all, 90 top left, center; 101 upper left, 158 bottom left, 168 right, 169 top right, 175 bottom left, 206 bottom right, 209 right, 226

City of Gaithersburg, Britta Monaco, pages 61 center right, 86 top left, 90 bottom, 93 right, 101 lower left, 102 bottom center, 173 top center, 206 upper right

Lani Harmon, pages 12 right, 14 right, 26 lower left, 32 bottom right, 34 bottom left, 61 upper left, upper right, lower left; 63 upper cluster: lower center; lower cluster: right; 84 left, 85 top right, lower left; 86 bottom right, 89 all, 90 top left, 93 left, 103 center left, 111 bottom, 112, 114 bottom left, bottom right; 117 bottom right, 133 bottom left, bottom right; 171 bottom right, 173 bottom left, 176 left, 181 left

Mark Harris, Frozentime Images Photography, frozentime.se, pages 16, 84 right, 87 all, 92 left, 98 left, 102 bottom right, 224

Elenor Hodges, page 204

iStock

    trekandshoot, page 118

    norcon, page 119 bottom left

    seven75, page 119 top

    MachineHeadz, page 124 bottom right

    JillianCain, page 130 top

    AmeeC, page 139

    HildeAnna, page 229 bottom right

    Gajus, page 226 top right

Jenn Lockwood, pages 9 left, 194

Melanie Meren, page 160 upper right

Katherine Pacelli, pages 9 right, 76, 77 bottom left, 145 bottom right, 195 upper right, 236 bottom right

Adam Segel-Moss, pages 68 bottom right, 73 top

Jennifer Shores and Gilbert Carmichael, pages 15, 50 right

Shutterstock/Wayne Via, page 230 top left

Rebecca Fox Stoddard and Andrew Stoddard, NurturingRoots.org, pages 28 bottom, 46, 50 left, 55 upper right, 58 bottom, 63 upper cluster: top center, lower cluster: center and bottom left; 68 left, 73 bottom, 74 all, 77 top left, bottom right; 99 top, 106 bottom left, 110 bottom left, 124 top center, bottom left; 125 upper left, bottom left; 134, 136, 143 all, 144 top, 145 top left, center left, bottom left; 149 center right, 150 upper and bottom left, 152 upper right, 158 bottom right, 161 center, 162 bottom, 163 top, 168 left, 169 top left, lower right; 170 all, 172–173 top left, 173 bottom right, 174–175 top left, 174 bottom left; 175 top center, top right, center, bottom right; 176 right, 179 all, 180 top right, lower right, bottom left; 181 bottom center, bottom right; 182 upper left, bottom left; 191 bottom left, bottom right; 207 upper right, 208 upper left, 236 bottom left

Kaia Twombly, page 55 bottom left

Wikimedia

Used under a Creative Commons Attribution-Share Alike CCAS 4.0 International license: Rhododendrites, page 177

Used under a Creative Commons Attribution-Share Alike CCAS 3.0 Unported license: Fungus Guy, page 119 bottom right

Used under a Creative Commons Attribution-Share Alike CCAS 2.0 Generic license: Oregon State University, page 137

ARTISTS AND DESIGNERS

Jim Calder, page 20 bottom right

Sharon Danks, page 27 upper right

Patrick Dougherty and Elsa Hoffman, page 14 left

EarlySpace, pages 12 right, 26 top left, top right, bottom left; 27 bottom right, 28 top left, top right; 32 bottom left and right, 33 center left, bottom left; 36 bottom, 39 upper right, 40 top, center, and bottom left; 41 center, 43, 53, 85 top left, top right; 89 lower right; 91 center, bottom left, bottom right; 98 bottom left, 101 all, 117 bottom right, 123 bottom right, 158 upper right, 160 all, 191 top left, top right

Earthplay, page 69 bottom right

Lan Hogue, pages 69 top left, 127 bottom left,

Meyer Design, pages 60 bottom left (sand wall), 61 upper left, 62, 127 center right

Natural Learning Initiative, page 39 bottom left

Ed Radvazzo, page 149 bottom right

Antje Schwabersberger and Henrik Hubner, pages 22 bottom left, 39 upper left, 102 bottom left

Suzy Scollon, page 72 all

Alyson Shotz, page 36 center left

SoundPlay.com, pages 23 top right, 50 right

Callie Warner, page 21 bottom left

Weenotes, page 50 bottom right

ILLUSTRATIONS

Nancy Striniste, page 217

All other illustrations by Jennifer Ren

LOCATIONS

Bender Jewish Community Center in Rockville, Maryland, pages 26 top right, 123 bottom right

Brookside Gardens, Wheaton, Maryland, page 189 bottom left

Burgundy Center for Wildlife Studies, Capon Bridge, West Virginia, page 151 top left, top right

Campbell Elementary School, Arlington, Virginia, pages 89 bottom left, 90 top left, 111 bottom, 117 bottom right

Chanticleer Garden in Wayne, Pennsylvania, page 33 top right, center right, bottom right; 102 center right

Children's Garden at Winterthur, Winterthur, Delaware, page 151 bottom right

Clarendon Child Care Center, Arlington, Virginia, page 132 bottom right, 190, 191 top left, top right

Cleveland Botanical Garden, Ohio, page 98 top right, 132 bottom left, 159 top

Coastal Maine Botanical Garden, Boothbay, Maine, page 32 top, 159 bottom

Constitution Gardens Park, Gaithersburg, Maryland, pages 36 bottom, 37, 41 center, 53, 85 top left, 90 bottom left, 91 top left, 101 all, 102 bottom center, 168 right, 226

Creative Minds International Public Charter School, Washington, DC, pages 40 bottom left, 43, 51 top left, 98 bottom left, 158 upper right, 162 center right

Drew Model Elementary School, Arlington, Virginia, pages 26 top left, 28 top left, 32 bottom left and right, 39 upper right

Green Spring Gardens, Alexandria, Virginia, page 22 upper left

Honeysuckle Tea House in Chapel Hill, North Carolina, pages 21 top right, 98 bottom right, 207 upper left

Irvine Nature Center, Owings Mills, Maryland, page 51 top right, bottom left

Ithaca Children's Garden, Ithaca, New York, page 39 bottom right

Longwood Gardens, Kennett Square, Pennsylvania, page 196 bottom left

Lowell School, Washington, DC, pages 60 bottom left, 85 top right, 89 lower right, 91 center, bottom left, bottom right; 111 center, 198 left

Luci and Ian Family Garden at the Lady Bird Johnson Wildflower Center, Austin, Texas, pages 152 bottom left, 196 top

Mondo Verde Public Charter School, Washington, DC, page 198 right

Montessori School of Northern Virginia, Annandale, Virginia, pages 28 top right, 40 top and center left, 61 top right, 103 center left, 113 bottom left, 127 center right, bottom right

Nurturing Roots School and Discover Woods, McLean, Virginia, pages 42, 106 bottom left, 124 bottom left, 134, 158 bottom right, 162 bottom, 168 left, 207 upper right

Otto Wels Elementary School, Berlin, Germany, pages 156–157 all, 188

River Farm (headquarters of American Horticultural Society), Alexandria, Virginia, page 67 bottom left

Thomas Jefferson Elementary School, Falls Church, Virginia, page 186 right

U.S. Botanic Garden, Washington, DC, page 34 top left

Washington Lee High School, Arlington, Virginia, pages 80, 81 top left, upper right; 127 top right

Westlawn Elementary, Falls Church, Virginia, page 189 top

INDEX

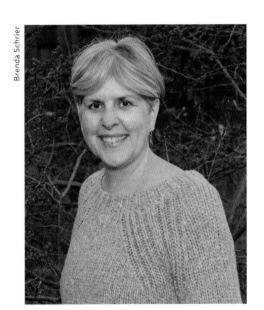

Brenda Schrier

Nancy Striniste is the founder and principal designer at EarlySpace, LLC. She has a background as both a landscape designer and an early childhood educator. She teaches at Antioch New England University in their Nature-based Early Childhood graduate certificate program and serves on the leadership team of NoVA Outside.

Nancy's goal is to bring nature to the places where children spend their time: backyards, schoolyards, churchyards, parks, and early childhood settings. She has worked with families, schools, childcare centers, municipalities, and organizations to create sustainably designed natural play and learning spaces and to teach about how to use the outdoors for learning and play.

Published in 2019 by Timber Press, Inc.

The Haseltine Building
133 S.W. Second Avenue, Suite 450
Portland, Oregon 97204-3527
timberpress.com

Printed in China

Text and cover design by Mary Winkelman Velgos

ISBN 978-1-60469-825-1

Catalog records for this book are available
from the Library of Congress and the British Library.

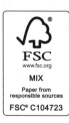

FSC
www.fsc.org
MIX
Paper from
responsible sources
FSC® C104723